"Stress is one of the biggest stumbling blocks to creating a life without alcohol. The challenge that Rebecca Williams skillfully tackles in her book, *Simple Ways to Unwind without Alcohol*, is learning to take the edge off our day with better habits. This approach brilliantly puts less emphasis on eliminating alcohol, and more on integrating new behaviors that basically crowd out drinking with healthy behavior changes with lasting impact."

> —**Kristen Manieri**, host of the *60 Mindful Minutes*
> podcast, and author of *Better Daily Mindfulness Habits*

"Post-pandemic, rebooting life mindfully back to health is a special gift. This is a complete guide to examining your inner and outer environments by slowing down, being compassionate to yourself, and becoming your own best friend. This 'coach' is evidence-based, yet an easy companion on the journey back from alcohol abuse. It is a collection of pithy advice to use throughout a year of building new habits."

> —**Pollyanna V. Casmar, PhD**, health sciences clinical
> professor at University of California, San Diego; and
> author of *Compassion Meditation for Trauma Group*
> (*CBCT-Vet*)

"*Simple Ways to Unwind without Alcohol* is wonderful life advice for anyone whether you are considering quitting drinking or not. Rebecca includes great tips for cultivating boundaries, making your living space tranquil, making connections at work, reducing stress, and more. It is highly organized with easy checklists. She anticipates questions about how to maneuver through your new journey without alcohol, and delivers real advice for a life well lived."

> —**Pamela Crane, MS, C-IAY**
> speaker, host of *The Yoga Pɾ*
> Interoceptive Performance

T0000866

"Rebecca Williams does a masterful job at compassionately guiding the sober-curious reader on how to change their relationship to alcohol. We are creatures of habit, and change is not always an easy thing to do. *Simple Ways to Unwind without Alcohol* opens a doorway for anyone who chooses to change by walking through this process, leading to a new life filled with freedom, healing, joy, and peace."

—**Steven Washington**, movement and wellness expert, author of *Recovering You*, and founder of SWE Studio

"The strategies in this book are deceptively simple but help to create a container of structure, clarity, and sanity. I noticed how many of these approaches have supported my own long-term sobriety, and I've continued to add to my self-care toolbox thanks to this fabulous book. You cannot go wrong with these practices."

—**Jenna Hollenstein**, **MS**, **RD**, nutrition therapist, and author of *Intuitive Eating for Life* and *Eat to Love*

"Changing is hard because we don't actually have much practice being our new self. Rebecca Williams, with this wonderful book, helps with the most important question about change: How do I actually do it? You never feel alone as she offers a how-to on such skills as new ways to be kind to yourself, how to talk to loved ones, and have fun. This book is a gem, and I can't wait to share it with my clients!"

—**Richard Brouillette**, **LCSW**, psychotherapist, *Psychology Today* blogger, and author of *Your Coping Skills Aren't Working*

Simple
Ways to
Unwind
without
Alcohol

**50 Tips to Drink Less
& Enjoy More**

Rebecca E. Williams, PhD

New Harbinger Publications, Inc.

Publisher's Note

Distributed in Canada by Raincoast Books

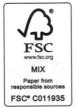

NEW HARBINGER PUBLICATIONS is a registered trademark of New Harbinger Publications, Inc.

Copyright © 2023 by Rebecca E. Williams
New Harbinger Publications, Inc.
5720 Shattuck Avenue
Oakland, CA 94609
www.newharbinger.com

Cover design by Sara Christian; Interior design by Michele Waters-Kermes; Acquired by Jennye Garibaldi; Edited by Kristi Hein

---

Library of Congress Cataloging-in-Publication Data on file

Printed in the United States of America

23   22   21

10   9   8   7   6   5   4   3   2   1   First Printing

"*Simple Ways to Unwind without Alcohol* is an easy-to-understand, easy-to-follow, and very strengths-based treasure chest of insightful and compassionate ways to self-soothe, which helps us to reduce feelings of shame and build true self-confidence. From mindfulness and acceptance, as well as cognitive behavioral therapy (CBT), Rebecca offers invaluable guidance on how to work with our tricky minds, and offer ourselves compassion to achieve our goals and choose a life without alcohol. This guide is a must-have resource!"

> **—Yuliana Gallegos Rodríguez, PhD**, assistant clinical professor at the University of California, San Diego School of Medicine; and clinical psychologist at the VA Medical Center

"This practical book provides enjoyable alternatives to alcohol, catering to various reasons for drinking. Its user-friendly table of contents makes it an easily accessible and valuable resource for all. With its engaging content, it's a book worth revisiting again and again."

> **—Denise G. Dempsey, CHT, MEd**, mindfulness-based stress reduction (MBSR) instructor, hypnotherapist, and author of *Mindfulness Meditations for Stress*

"What a gift! Or more accurately, what a treasure trove of gifts! The author's expertise and engaging and encouraging approach shine throughout the book as she guides us through each strategy with clear, concise, and easy-to-understand instructions. The emphasis on scientific backing provides readers with confidence in the efficacy of the methods presented. This is now one of my go-to recommendations for loved ones and clients!"

> **—Carolyn B. Allard, PhD, ABPP**, professor, and director of the clinical psychology PhD program at Alliant International University; and author of *Trauma Informed Guilt Reduction Therapy*

For those who have made the bold decision to redirect their energy away from alcohol toward an empowered new beginning.

Contents

Introduction   1

Chapter 1   Soothe Your Mind   7

  1. Meditate, But Keep It Short and Sweet   9

  2. Open Up to Breathing   12

  3. Befriend Your Inner Therapist   14

  4. Notice Your Emotions; Trust Your Intuition   16

  5. Create a Social Media and News Detox   18

Chapter 2   Engage with Your Body   23

  6. Refresh with Sleep and Rest   25

  7. Restore Yourself with Yoga   28

  8. Hydrate for Health   31

  9. Walk It Off   33

  10. Choose Mindful Bodywork   35

Chapter 3   Love Your Home   39

  11. Learn Feng Shui Tips   41

  12. Declutter with Kindness   44

  13. Clean with the Music On   47

  14. Make Friends with Your Chores   50

  15. Claim Your Corner Spot   52

Chapter 4   Rediscover Nature   56

  16. Cultivate Your Indoor Sanctuary   59

  17. Enjoy Your Outdoor Oasis   61

  18. Explore Nature Trails   63

  19. Write or Draw for Growth   65

  20. Watch Your Nature   68

Chapter 5   Nurture Your Relationships   72

  21. Embrace New Communication Skills   74

  22. Renegotiate for Healing   77

  23. Schedule Your Down Time   79

  24. Rebuild Old and New Friendships   81

  25. Explore New Ways to Have Fun   84

Chapter 6   Reconnect with Your Work   90

  26. Build Boundaries for Wellness   92

  27. Make Your Home Work for Work   94

  28. Reclaim Your Work Friends   98

  29. Give Your Desk a Little Love   100

  30. Boss Yourself Around   102

Chapter 7   Savor Your Food and Drink   106

  31. Reignite Your Nutrition   108

  32. Celebrate Small Changes   111

  33. Plan Your Shopping and Prep   113

  34. Explore the Vegetarian Approach   116

  35. Be Mocktail Curious   119

Chapter 8 **Embrace Your Family**   **124**

   36. Start Where You Are   **126**

   37. Rebuild Connections with Kids   **129**

   38. Offer Kindness to Elders   **132**

   39. Bond with Animals   **135**

   40. Take Small Breaks to Recharge   **138**

Chapter 9 **Respect Your Money**   **142**

   41. Review Your Finances with Love   **144**

   42. Decrease Spending Today   **148**

   43. Pay Off Debt and Save   **151**

   44. Learn to Earn   **153**

   45. Plan Low-Cost or No-Cost Fun   **156**

Chapter 10 **Celebrate Your Spirit**   **160**

   46. Rebalance in the Here and Now   **162**

   47. Get Your Art On   **164**

   48. Engage in Mutual Support   **167**

   49. Give Back–A Little Goes a Long Way   **170**

   50. Find Joy in Everyday Moments   **174**

Notes of Gratitude   **178**

Resources   **180**

References   **185**

Introduction

If you've been thinking of taking a break from alcohol or stopping drinking altogether, this little book might just give you the inspiration you need. I don't want to complicate things. Life is already pretty full as it is. I simply offer you an opportunity to explore ways to unwind and take care of yourself without alcohol.

There is no quick fix or one size fits all. This is a personal decision only you can make and a choice only you can return to each day. No big parades, no balloons, no greeting cards. This is, surprisingly, a quiet decision. One that reconnects you to who you want to be today. There will be no judgment of past behaviors or dwelling on past regrets. Those are not important right now. What is important is your ability to reclaim your calm mind, reenergize your body, and renew your relationships.

NOTE: If you believe you have a severe addiction to alcohol, this may not be the book for you right now. Getting professional help would be your best bet.

This book is designed for you if you've had a nagging suspicion that alcohol, although great sometimes and a real social lubricant, is no longer something you want in your daily life. You may want to take a break to reevaluate your relationship to alcohol and see what you can discover without alcohol in your life. Or you may want to make a long-term shift. If you've been feeling out of balance, moody, agitated, disconnected, and disorganized, I think you will find a few gems here.

Alcohol use has increased, due to the unknowns of the COVID-19 pandemic (Acuff, Strickland, Tucker, and Murphy 2022) and other national and international stresses. People who drink to cope, and those who have current anxiety and depression, were more likely to report increased alcohol use (Capasso et al. 2021).

There is no perfect way to stop drinking; there is just *your* way. If you've been beating yourself up for failed efforts to stop, and thinking about, obsessing over, or reaching for alcohol: This is normal. Habits are, by definition, hard to give up. *Be kind to yourself.* Be forgiving of your behaviors. I wrote this book with your best interests in mind.

Read a few pages and reflect on how you're feeling. I encourage you to *breathe* throughout the book and throughout your day, especially when things get tough, when you feel exhausted, and when you feel tested. You'll find tips and strategies you can try every day or pick one to focus on for the week.

Each of the ten chapters targets an area of your life that may need your special attention as you change your relationship with alcohol, with specific recommendations for you to move a little further into your healing. The focus is on unwinding from stress and bringing comfort to your day without reaching for alcohol. We will explore ways to soothe your mind, engage with your body, love your home, rediscover nature, nurture your relationships, reconnect with your work life, savor your food and drink, embrace your family, respect your money, and celebrate your spirit. Each of these life areas has a particular connection to living without alcohol, and we will discover them step by step and day by day.

You may notice interesting links between the chapter topics and how you feel. Be curious about the parts of you that may have been buried beneath trying to cope with daily stressors. I have faith in you.

I know you can move through your day without alcohol, and I know now might be just the right time to try.

How to Get the Most from This Book

To get the most out of this book, use the strategies that make the most sense to you, leaving the rest for another time.

Slow and steady. This book is custom designed to offer you a fresh way to see yourself, experience your relationships, and engage in your environment now that you've decided to take a break from drinking alcohol. You can read and put into practice one topic per week, in order, and enjoy the small changes you make each month or for the whole year. Or you can skip to the topics that are most interesting and start there. Take your time and savor all of your successes.

Keep a journal. The benefits of writing are incredible. Journaling can lift your mood, improve your sense of well-being, and lessen your worrying. When you write how you're feeling and doing without alcohol, you will be surprised at what pops up. Commonly, *anxiety* may be one of the first emotions you feel. This is normal stuff. Write without judgment. Allow ten minutes of uninterrupted time daily to jot down what is on your mind.

Stay connected. You may tend to hide from others, out of fear or frustration. Or you may just not know what to do with yourself now that you've decided not to drink. This makes sense: You're letting a part of yourself go and may not yet know the new you. Remember to connect with people who are supportive. It may be just *one* caring person at the beginning of this journey. Small, heartfelt connections will certainly enhance the work you're doing as you read this book.

Quiet time. Before you embark on a topic in this book, take a few minutes of quiet for yourself, to prepare for what you're about to start. After completing your work on a soothing topic, take another few minutes to notice how you feel. This experience will be especially powerful when you change your drinking habits and interact with others. You're developing a new relationship with yourself and with others. Respect the changes you're making, and hold the space for yourself to get unstuck and heal.

Connect with a resource. If you want to dig a bit deeper into one of these topics, I have included a curated list of resources at the end of the book for you. Explore.

Seek help if you need to. For some, not drinking may be an easy decision and things may go smoothly. For others, there may be significant bumps in the road. If the ups and downs are a little too much for you to handle, reach out and get help from a compassionate, licensed mental health professional. You'll be surprised how that little extra help can make a big difference in your commitment to taking care of yourself.

Give yourself a chance to experience your days without alcohol. Begin to notice how your mind and body feel. Don't strain. If you get stuck, come back to this book for guidance, new ideas, or a bit of encouragement. What happens next is up to you. You deserve to be well.

Let Me Introduce Myself

I'm truly honored that you've decided to bring me along on your journey. A bit about me. I have been a psychologist for over twenty years and am coauthor of two popular books on mindfulness and addiction recovery. I've worked as a psychologist at a busy VA hospital, enjoyed a private practice, been a consultant on research projects, supervised psychology post-doctoral students, and taught graduate students pursuing a degree in marriage and family therapy. I'm also a yoga and meditation devotee; I taught yoga for fifteen years along the coast in beautiful La Jolla, California. But it wasn't always blue skies and palm trees for me. I grew up in the Bronx, New York. My family struggled with alcohol problems almost all of my life. I always thought we all needed some type of support, but we *never* got it. So I dedicated my life to understanding healing from the inside out. I know what works for deep well-being, and I know that most of us get stuck somewhere along the way.

The Journey Ahead

There are two important questions I want you to come back to as you read. The questions are custom designed for the topics you will be focusing on. They'll help you recenter yourself when things get rocky (we all know sometimes they will).

FIRST: What can I offer myself today?

Answer this heartfelt question when you feel unsure, angry, resentful, lonely, bored, or misunderstood—in other words, at some point in your day, every day.

SECOND: What can I let go of today?

Answer this powerful question when you feel burdened, overwhelmed, stiff, cranky, or forgetful—in other words, at some point in your day, every day.

You're catching on to what I think you might need as you navigate the ups and downs of your decision not to drink. Each day your answers will be different.

Rather than guessing, or asking someone else what they think you need or what you can let go of, answer these questions for yourself, honestly, as they relate to your emotional, physical, and spiritual well-being. What are you willing to offer yourself to gain that sense of calm? And what would you be willing to let go of in service of your healthy self? Once you get the hang of asking yourself these two vital questions at the end of each chapter, it will start to feel enjoyable. You will feel lighter. Especially when you offer yourself precisely what you need and let go of exactly what doesn't serve you.

There will be a brief checklist at the end of each chapter to keep things on track and to remind you which specific areas you'd like to focus on for the week.

Healing takes time and patience. That is what I wish for you. Give yourself time, and be patient. And *trust*. Trust that you're strong enough to take this next step and the step after that. Remember to give yourself moments to pause, reflect, and enjoy each day. Remember to *breathe*.

Chapter 1

Soothe Your Mind

All that you are seeking is also seeking you. If you sit still, it will find you. It has been waiting for you a long time.

—Clarissa Pinkola Estes

IN A BOOK ABOUT SIMPLE WAYS TO UNWIND without alcohol, I could have started chapter 1 with any way to soothe yourself. Which way gets the coveted number-one spot? I choose the mind first, not just because I am a psychologist and deeply believe in the importance of finding creative ways to take care of your mind, but because alcohol has a way of disrupting how your mind works. Alcohol affects your decision making and your mood. Alcohol impacts how your brain actually does what it's supposed to do. I wanted to start us on this journey with a profound admiration of our ability to feel better and make good decisions.

Let's entertain the possibility of being less reactive to daily stressors and more focused on what feels right. The goal is to cultivate the ability to create a calm and balanced mind. It takes practice and patience. It takes kindness and a light touch. I know you are worth it.

Let's start with the value of short meditations, then learn how to open up to breathing, to befriend your inner therapist, to notice your emotions but trust your intuition, and finally, to give yourself a mini break from the buzz of social media and news. All of this to prioritize your psychological health and build emotional resilience. This is the entry point. Ready to get started?

1. Meditate, But Keep It Short and Sweet

Of all the books, apps, podcasts, and YouTube videos out there on meditation, it comes down to this one thing. *Sit.* That's it. And because you may have been using alcohol to escape from your racing thoughts and kaleidoscope of feelings, just sitting quietly may be the last thing you want to do. I get it. When I first started meditating, I bought the fancy (and expensive) cushions, found the perfect spot in my house, and set aside the ideal time to "meditate." I proceeded to bring my coffee, a bowl of cereal, a newspaper (this was twenty years ago, when newspapers were a thing), and a very long to-do list with me to my fancy new meditation spot. I proceeded to distract myself, fidget, plan, and do just about everything but sit quietly. It took me and my bouncy mind a long time to settle down.

So, if you're anything like me, you've already tried meditation and think that you failed. Well, there is no failure in meditation. The only thing to do is stick with it. Even when you don't feel like it— *especially* when you don't feel like it. Your mind will look for any excuse to run, jump, and scramble out of it. That is normal.

We are looking for just *five minutes* a day. Find out what works best for you (first thing in the morning works best for me). Once you have a handle on your five minutes a day, you may go up to ten minutes a day. You can use a guided meditation, soft music, nature sounds, or just plain old silence. You can sit in a chair, on a cushion or blanket on the floor, or even start lying down.

There are so many benefits to even a short meditation for your emotional and physical health, it's the ideal place to start. Mediation can also help you continue your journey of not drinking. Top of the list is helping you manage stressful days. Some of that stress may have the added layer of intense cravings to drink alcohol. Meditation will help ease those cravings and calm your mind. The discipline of finding time each day to meditate will also help you become more patient with yourself. And meditating will give you the added benefit of accepting yourself and your experiences as they are. It's all about reclaiming the here and now. Mejia and Spann (2022) note these mental and physical benefits of adding short meditations to your day:

- Reduces your stress levels

- Helps you manage your day-to-day worried or sad feelings

- Lowers your blood pressure

- Improves your immune system

- Strengthens your memory

- Helps regulate your mood

- Improves your self-awareness

- Helps with your sleep

- Gives you a better chance not to return to drinking or other habits you'd like to stop.

These benefits happen over time, so stick with your meditation practice and notice whether you experience any of these important mood and health benefits. *Breathe.* Because you've just given up alcohol, meditation may feel weird, and your mind may be overly jumpy. It gets easier, I promise. Add a simple, short meditation time to your day and make it easy on yourself. That's it for now.

2. Open Up to Breathing

Remember, we are going to keep things delightfully simple here. Notice how I just snuck in the word *breathe* in tip #1? Let's focus on this a bit more. Of course, breathing comes naturally to us. But most of us take short, shallow breaths. Especially when we are anxious, worried, or fearful. Most of us breathe into our throat and chest and back out again, quickly in and quickly out.

Right now, try taking a long, slow, deep breath down into your belly. Good. Take another long, slow, deep breath. Great. One more, please. Feel the difference between your short shallow breath and your long deep breath? I want to reintroduce you to your own calming breath.

There are lots of documented benefits of a regular practice of simple, deep breathing. This type of belly breathing can calm your mind, slow down your thoughts, and allow you time to make good decisions for your health and well-being. If you get in a bind and are unsure what to do as it relates to drinking alcohol, you have permission to return to your long, slow, deep breathing. For instance, if you're at a special event with lots of alcohol flowing freely, before you make any decision, return to your long, slow, deep breathing practice. Or if you're with family members and are feeling stressed or frustrated, instead of reaching for a glass of wine or a beer to numb your feelings, pause a moment. Return to your breathing practice. Then make the next good decision.

It's also a great idea to bring this type of breathing into the five-minute daily meditation that you've started. If your mind starts to wonder (which it will, I guarantee), return to your long, slow, deep breathing. Here's how:

- Put both hands on your belly.

- Let the breath move down into your belly.

- Inhale and allow your belly to rise.

- Pause

- Exhale, allowing your belly to fall.

- Pause.

- Repeat.

Start with eight deep breaths each day. And if you get in a muddle at work or at home, practice two or three deep, healthy breaths before you make your next move, reply to your next email, or answer the next question someone throws your way. When you're not drinking, you might feel more tense than usual. This is part of the journey. In the past, you took care of that tension with alcohol (or looked forward to managing that tension with alcohol later in the day). Now you're learning new, simple ways to take care of your mind and emotions. Breathing signals your nervous system to calm down and reset. And what better way to tackle that next stressor that comes your way?

3. Befriend Your Inner Therapist

I am a therapist, so of course I'm a huge fan of seeing a therapist if and when you can, to tackle some of those thorny issues. However, not everyone has the resources. Or perhaps you'd like to have a plan in place between therapy sessions. What would it be like to have an awesome therapist inside your mind who gave you gentle support and guidance every single day? Someone filled with kindness and compassion for you and your journey toward emotional wellness without turning to alcohol? Someone who is *really* in your corner?

Well, good news! You have access to that inner therapist right now. That inner therapist is there with you each day when you make your decision not to drink. Whether you're out with friends, or home after a long day at work, or needing a break from your kids (or all of the above!), your inner therapist is there for you. Your inner therapist is understanding and encouraging; they get what you're going through. Your inner therapist listens and treats you exactly how your best friend in the world would treat you when you're going through a rough time or feeling unsure.

Instead of bullying yourself or tightening the grip of negative comments around yourself, what would it feel like to be big-hearted toward yourself? *Breathe.* This big-hearted feeling toward yourself is called *self-compassion.* Quite a few researchers are studying the benefits of self-compassion and coping in stressful or demanding situations (Ewert, Vater, and Schröder-Abé 2021). Introducing self-compassion into your life on a steady basis will greatly improve your ability to mindfully cope with the day-to-day stress that we all experience. And since many people drink alcohol to cope with stress, it's nice to know that activating this compassionate inner therapist actually works to settle your mind down and manage what is in front of you.

Here are a few simple techniques to call forth your inner therapist; try doing them in order:

1. Give yourself a few moments to get quiet and focus on your breath.

2. Ask yourself: *What support do I need right now?*

3. Listen to the answer that comes up for you.

4. Offer yourself words of encouragement, such as *I am focusing on my mental health today* or *I have the strength to get through this situation today* or *Being kind to myself always feels like the right thing to do.*

5. Follow through with giving yourself the support you need.

6. Repeat these steps whenever your emotional life needs tending to. (Hint: This may be an everyday practice.)

So when you get in a jam or have a hard time making the best decision, get quiet, activate your inner therapist, and follow the intelligent advice you receive. You might notice that your big-heartedness expands outward to include those around you. What a wonderful way to move through the world!

4. Notice Your Emotions; Trust Your Intuition

Most of us can recognize the shape of our emotions. Fear, hurt, anger, sadness, rage, envy, boredom, happiness, or joy, to name just a few. These human emotions are part of our everyday life; *nobody* gets through life without experiencing them. It's important to recognize your intense feelings but not attach to them. Especially when it comes to feelings around drinking alcohol. Drinking to cope with any particularly intense feeling—like anger, despair, or anxiety—can lead you down a dark alley, a scary place where you may not be able to see a safe way back to the lighted path. Drinking, at the beginning, may feel like it lights the path for you. But over time, alcohol might make things worse, and when emotions feel overwhelming, you can lose sight of what you really want and need. But there is a way back.

Let's talk about your *intuition*—which is incredibly powerful, although perhaps less understood than your emotions. Your intuition is that *gut feeling* that something is right or wrong. We all have it. It comes from that *truth* inside of you (Chestney 2020). Your intuition doesn't come from other people's judgment of you and what you should or shouldn't do. There are plenty of other people's opinions to go around; though well-intentioned at times, they're usually not very helpful. Many opinions on social media come from people you don't know, who don't know you. Intuition is a perfect partner when you're deciding not to drink, because it guides you to make high-level decisions for your emotional well-being and health.

If you've ever had the feeling that something just doesn't feel right when meeting someone, going somewhere, or doing something, that is your intuition trying to get your attention (and possibly save you from a dangerous situation). It's not exactly scientific. Intuition bypasses your brain and heads right to your gut. Instead of ignoring or shrugging off that weird feeling, start listening to it.

Your thoughts and experience with alcohol will change when you begin to listen to, trust, and act on your intuition. When you were drinking alcohol, your intuition may have been blunted or just too quiet for you to hear. Now you have the opportunity to reengage with that part of you that holds deep knowledge about what is right for you. Intuition is an inside job. Try these simple steps to practice listening to your intuition:

1. Before making a decision, ask yourself: *What is the right thing for me to do at this moment?*

2. Sometimes, rather than jumping in with both feet, pausing or doing nothing may be the right thing

3. Intuition helps clarify and guide you, allow it do what it is designed to do.

4. Reflect back on the experience of listening to your intuition: How did things turn out for you?

Trust your intuition and give it a chance to blossom as you travel on your curious journey of not drinking.

5. Create a Social Media and News Detox

Most of us spend about two and a half hours on social media every day; some end up spending over three hours daily scrolling through the (usually bad) news. Of course, social media has lots of positive facets, including connecting with friends, targeting job prospects, building your business, following people you admire, or keeping up with current events. News keeps us informed about what is going on nationally and internationally. However, all that social media and news consumption may have a shadow side for your mental well-being.

Constantly comparing yourself to others is not how things are meant to be for your healthy mind. In fact, a Finnish psychologist's research suggested that for true happiness, it's better to set your own standard, instead of comparing yourself to others (Martela, 2020).

Some people find it difficult or stressful to look at photos of other people drinking and partying when they are choosing to abstain from alcohol, especially at the beginning of the journey. And since reducing stress is the point, detoxing from social media may be positive not just for your mood but also for reducing your alcohol consumption.

An onslaught of bad news can put anyone in a negative feedback loop that's hard to shake. A bunch of new research shows that a diet of incessant social media and news can negatively impact our mind and moods (Boukes and Vliegenthart 2017). And as you stop drinking, you need to take special care to nourish your mind with positive experiences to avoid depression and anxiety. This may sound radical, but in your search for small ways to soothe your mind, see if decreasing your time on social media has a positive effect on your emotional health.

Sounds good in theory, but how does this work? Detoxing from social media or news means just giving yourself a set period of staying off the platforms and apps. You might be thinking *I'm already giving up alcohol; why should I give up one of my other pleasures? Breathe.* Here are a few of the benefits; see if any of these would be helpful for you right now:

- You will improve your ability to focus on one task at a time.

- You will have more time for yourself.

- You will have more time for your family and friends (actually in person, rather than on a screen).

- You may even notice an immediate boost in your mood.

When you're not relying on alcohol for a temporary mood fix, these benefits will have a real impact on your overall well-being. When you're not drinking, you may find it easier to detox from social media and the news because your mind is clearer, and you will naturally gravitate to taking better care of yourself and your mind. Taking a conscious break from social media could even amplify the positive effects of lower or no alcohol consumption. Make it easy on yourself and give this soothing technique a go.

Try these simple steps to begin to reclaim your calm:

1. Choose an amount of time you plan to detox (one day, one weekend, one week, or one month),

2. Delete or pause your social media and news apps (don't worry, you can reinstall them later).

3. Let your close friends and family know you will be off line, and let them know how long that will be.

4. Decide what you will do with the extra two to three hours each day.

5. Replace negative input with encouraging input to improve your mood.

Check in with yourself on how you're feeling. After the first moments (or days) of agitation and impulses to check, is your mind beginning to cool down? Note: Some of the soothing suggestions in this book are fun and healthy ways to use your newfound extra time.

● ● ● ● ●

Let's revisit those two reflection questions from the introduction and focus on them when soothing your mind. Take a few moments to honestly answer:

What can I offer my mind today?

What can I let go of in my mind today?

Soothe Your Mind Checklist

How have you decided to soothe your mind so that you can feel that sense of calm without reaching for, or thinking about, alcohol? Read through this checklist and choose one area to focus on this week for a healthy and less-stressed mind:

- ☐ Carve out five minutes for a quiet meditation a few times this week.

- ☐ Practice long, slow, deep breaths three times a day to calm yourself down.

- ☐ Take the time to befriend your inner therapist once each day to support your well-being.

- ☐ Learn to trust your intuition one time this week and use it as a guide for quality life decisions.

- ☐ Plan for a social media and news detox within the next week.

Now that you've taken a look at some of the ways to soothe your mind, we'll venture into ways to engage with your body without alcohol. You are on the right track; keep going.

Chapter 2

Engage with Your Body

Our body reveals who we are. Through this awareness, we enter the path of practice.

—Pat Phalen

I WANT YOU TO FORGET ABOUT DOING (or not doing) exercise for a moment. Forget about the fact that you were an athlete in high school, or that you've always been awkward at exercising, or that you hate sports in general. This next phase of your life is about healing and movement. It's about getting reacquainted with your body in a soothing, comfortable way, now that you're shifting your relationship with drinking. This means neither taking your body to its limit nor putting your head in the sand about your fitness and ignoring it altogether. There is a place somewhere in the middle that feels right for you.

Your health and fitness may look totally different now from what you once thought—or hoped—it would be. But I guarantee you, taking a fresh look at how your body feels and functions will be extremely helpful as you navigate this time in your life without alcohol. Most important, try your best not to be hard on yourself.

Getting to know your body again, in a new way, is a listening game. Now that your drinking habits have changed, listen to what your body needs. You might be surprised that your body has different needs now. You might find yourself gravitating to things that are more restorative and slower-paced. Once you start listening, you might notice that physically slowing down is the beginning of healing. Especially if you've been going at a high speed for the past few years. *Breathe*. Spend some time refreshing with sleep and rest, restoring with yoga, hydrating for health, walking off the stress, and choosing healing bodywork. Listen and begin.

6. Refresh with Sleep and Rest

How is your sleep? No, really: How do you sleep? On a scale from one to ten, with one being terrible sleep and ten being wonderful sleep, where does yours fall? Most people who drink alcohol regularly report poor sleep. Even small amounts of alcohol can have a significant impact. Research confirms this. Although alcohol has a mild relaxing effect, the type of sleep you were getting was most likely restless and disturbed, especially from about two in the morning onward. That's when alcohol's relaxing effect starts to wear off. It's no surprise if you're also taking prescribed or over-the-counter sleeping medication to help you get a good night's sleep. If you have been waking up multiple times a night, not able to get back to sleep, or just feeling exhausted in the morning (or all day), alcohol may be the culprit. Once you stop or reduce drinking, it may take a little while for your sleep to get back to a normal rhythm. Don't panic if you continue to have some restless nights. Your body needs time to heal and find its way back to a normal sleep cycle. *Breathe*. Now let's develop a fresh new sleep routine.

Start with setting up your bedroom as the soothing sanctuary you deserve. Try a few of these respectful sleep healing techniques. Pick any one to start with.

- **No TV and no work in the bedroom.** If you're used to bingeing on your favorite crime drama or bringing your work to bed with you, this would be a great time to give yourself a boundary to support a deeply relaxing bedroom.

- **No scrolling one hour before bedtime.** If you're accustomed to mindlessly looking at your phone in bed, would you be willing to give yourself an hour's reprieve before lights out, to offer your mind a chance to rest?

- **Clean up any clutter in your bedroom.** Letting your mind and eyes relax after a long day is important for unwinding. Start with picking up any clutter on the floor and work your way up to removing anything on your bedroom chairs, dresser, and bed.

- **Add fresh sheets.** Give yourself permission to buy a new set of sheets to signal this new phase of better sleep. If you can't afford a set of sheets just now, spray a scented, nonaerosol spray with a calming fragrance, like lavender, around your bedroom in the evening or use your favorite essential oils in a diffuser one hour before turning out the lights.

- **Make your bedroom darker and cooler.** Use shades or curtains, and modify your sleepwear or blankets to give your body a chance to cool down throughout the night.

- **Get in a rhythm of a regular bedtime every night.** A consistent bedtime will alert your mind and body that it's time to shut down and prepare for sleep. Most people find that with a regular routine they wake up earlier and more refreshed, without the hassle of a hangover.

- **Enjoy a cup of comforting herbal tea one hour before your bedtime.** Just as adding a relaxing scent to your bedroom signals that it is time to relax, herbal tea offers your mind that same signal. It's common wisdom among herbalists that chamomile, lavender, valerian root, and passionflower teas offer the best support for relaxing at bedtime.

Getting into a routine with a few simple habits will help over the days and weeks ahead. Take care of yourself like you're taking care of a toddler who's had a very active day. What does that toddler (in you) need for a calm sleep? Give yourself that special care, beginning tonight.

Most people think *rest* is just another word for sleep. But as you go through your days without alcohol, rest is going to be your new best friend. You've probably relied on alcohol to switch off after a full day or to manage burnout. Without alcohol, you may find yourself struggling to power down. This is where rest comes in—in finding quiet, uninterrupted moments in your day. Rest can be closing your eyes at your desk for five minutes or taking a break and lying down at home with a covering over your eyes for twenty minutes. Perhaps for you it's taking a bath, stretching, caring for your plants, reading a few pages of your favorite book, or listening to tranquil music. Or rest could be getting outside and taking five long, slow, deep breaths and looking at the clouds in the sky. Find a few minutes each day for your personal rest period, to recharge and reclaim a calmer mind and body.

Decide which of these simple rest activities will work best for you and which you can do regularly. Physical rest includes slowing down and pausing your physical activities for a short time each day. The trick is that to really soothe yourself (and your central nervous system), you need to take rest seriously and find creative ways to incorporate it into your healing life.

7. Restore Yourself with Yoga

There is a good chance you've tried yoga either online at home or at your local yoga studio or neighborhood gym. If you haven't yet, it may be a good idea to give yoga a try now that you're taking a break from alcohol. Both online and local studios offer free or low-cost introductory classes to get the ball rolling. As you change your drinking habits, yoga can provide the comprehensive support your body needs (Walia et al. 2021). According to the Johns Hopkins School of Medicine (2023), among its many important benefits, yoga has been shown to:

- Enhance your strength and flexibility

- Improve your balance

- Ease your back pain and arthritis

- Help your heart health

- Support your sleep

- Lift your mood

- Manage your stress

- Link you up with a caring community

- Improve your self-care

I don't think about these benefits when I do yoga. It just makes me feel better, and that helps me move through the day a little easier.

As you cut down or quit drinking, do you think you might get a little extra boost from yoga too? As you move deeper into engaging with your body, focus on trying slower types of yoga like restorative yoga or yin yoga. (Of course, check in with your doctor before starting any exercise program.)

If you've already been doing yoga for a while, I suggest taking a restorative yoga class now that you're exploring sobriety. Many yoga instructors recommend that even advanced yoga students take beginning restorative classes. At first it may feel like you're going back to the basics and it's too slow or too boring. *Perfect.* That's exactly what your healing body and brain need now—the slower the better.

Many authors write that before they decided to try restorative yoga they experienced a medical or mental health crisis or had become buried in burnout (Raheem 2022). But you don't have to hit the wall before benefiting from restorative yoga.

To learn more about restorative yoga, look into the classes on gaia.com to see if it's the right fit for you. To find a class near you (whether you're home or away from home), check the largest online directory, https://yogafinder.com.

Your brain and body will be changing as you remove alcohol from your days, and it's important to create a safe space for you to change and heal.

Restorative yoga also creates space to feel your inner quietness without all the loudness and busyness of the outside world. Restorative yoga classes are especially helpful for recovering from long-term effects of COVID-19 or other respiratory conditions—indeed, any illness or injury—or from post-traumatic stress or other significant life stressors. But you needn't wait for a crisis to find a restorative class to start incorporating this type of healing activity into your life.

Many of the restorative exercises can even be done on your bed in the morning or before you end your day. Restorative yoga is usually helpful for all body types, all ages, and wherever you are on your journey of healing. You deserve to reconnect with your body in a new, slower, more patient way.

8. Hydrate for Health

You might be surprised to learn of all the benefits of hydrating yourself. Many of us are dehydrated, and this is especially likely if you've been drinking alcohol regularly. You've probably heard that alcohol is a diuretic—when you drink it, your body processes fluids faster. You may have experienced periods of dehydration without even knowing it. Fortunately, getting back to drinking a healthy amount of water is pretty easy (and not expensive).

The many incredible benefits you can expect from staying hydrated (National Council on Aging 2021; Silver 2020) include:

- Improving how your brain works, including steadying your emotions and managing anxiety—both are crucial, since emotional instability and anxiety are common concerns when you get sober.

- Improving your digestion, which is important, since alcohol can wreak havoc on your gut health. Your gut and brain are connected physically through millions of nerve cells; thus gut health affects your brain health.

- Boosting energy levels—it's common to need a bit more energy when changing your relationship with alcohol.

- Easing joint pain. Lessening of aches and pains is always welcome, especially when changing your physical health.

- Improving your temperature regulation. Have you noticed alcohol tends to make you feel uncomfortably warm? Drinking more water helps you cool down when you're dehydrated.

- Improving your bladder health. Alcohol can irritate the bladder and exacerbate potential urinary tract infections; water helps flush harmful bacteria from the bladder and keep UTIs at bay.

- Easing headaches. Especially if you've struggled with headaches or migraines related to drinking alcohol, you may find that hydration prevents these debilitating headaches.

- Decreasing early aging and the risk of chronic disease. A recent study found that adults who are not properly hydrated may age faster and face a higher risk of chronic diseases (National Institutes of Health 2023).

Even if you enjoy just one of these benefits as you change your hydration habits, it could mean a wonderful improvement in your overall health and your mood. Think of water as a good, supportive friend on your journey.

I'm asking you to add just one glass of water per day and check in with how you feel physically and emotionally. *Breathe.* Keep water with you at work, when you're out, in your car, and at home or in your home office. Take a break from reading this right now, grab a glass of water, and take a good drink. Great! When you're going out to eat with friends and family, ask for water every time (if it's not brought to your table). I know this may seem simple, but give it a try. Reach for water to soothe your body, decrease the effects of dehydration now that you're alcohol-free, and continue on your healing journey.

9. Walk It Off

Although most any form of exercise will be good for you in your focus on your healthy sobriety, one of the most important is the simple act of walking. Most of us can fit walking into our day. It doesn't have to be miles and miles—you don't need to start training to run a marathon or half-marathon (as cool as that sounds). I'm talking about starting with a fifteen- to twenty-minute walk each day—around your neighborhood or on your lunch break at work, or after work before it gets too dark outside, with a friend or partner or with your kids.

If you commit to short walks each day, you will be giving yourself little rewards for both your body and mind. Walking can offer time for reflection and can ease your stress. If you now have long evenings without alcohol, walking might be just the ticket to fill your time with something soothing. The added benefit is the positive interactions you will have with your environment.

Are you thinking *I've got too much to do—how is this going to help me unwind?* Or *I used to be an athlete—how is a short walk going to get me back in shape?* This is not about getting back in shape. Walking to unwind is different. Walking has a ton of health benefits, and now that you're not drinking alcohol, which one (or more) of these benefits would resonate with you right now? Much research has shown (as outlined on healthline.com; Chertoff 2016) that adding walking to your day will help you:

- Burn calories

- Strengthen your heart

- Lower your blood sugar

- Ease any joint pain

- Boost your immune function

- Increase your energy

- Improve your mood

- Tone your legs

- Enhance your creative thinking

Even if you just want to boost your immune function and not worry about any of the other benefits right now, you're definitely going in the right direction. The key is to *make it easy* and make it a regular part of each week.

So get your walking gear ready this evening and prepare to hit the pavement or trail tomorrow. You can enjoy your walk taking in the sounds around you, or bring your earbuds and favorite music, book, or podcast, or find a walking buddy or group to share the experience. Connect your walking time with who you are: someone exploring a sober lifestyle, find the joy in each step along the way. If you miss a day, begin anew the next day. Happy walking!

10. Choose Mindful Bodywork

Not drinking alcohol can be uncomfortable if you've been accustomed to drinking regularly. That's why giving yourself new ways to feel better is so important. I used to think getting a massage or going to the chiropractor was a special event, done only a few times a year, if at all. It never occurred to me that getting regular bodywork was part of my overall health care. Things have changed for me since I made a commitment to my overall well-being. Bodywork is health care. That's how we have to think of any bodywork. If your shoulders ache, or your back is always stiff, or your head pounds with a weekly headache, now is the time to listen to what your body needs and take care of yourself on a deeper level.

Explore what body healing options are available to you, and set aside time and money to take care of your body. For example, if a monthly massage costs around $90 (including a tip) for a one-hour session, that is about $3 per day for a month. Is there something you can give up so you can move that daily $3 over to your personal health care account? Oh, that's right, you've already given up an expensive habit—can you move the money you spent on drinks over to your health care basket? If you're not ready for a full hour massage, please give yourself the gift of a half-hour massage.

If you've never had a massage in the context of not drinking, you may experience both a physical and an emotional release this time around. There may be lots of pent-up tension you didn't even realize was there. Give your body time to acclimate to these new healing practices. If you have a history of childhood trauma or a recent traumatic experience, proceed slowly, always with a trusted and licensed health practitioner. Ask the practitioner to massage just your feet or just your neck. If you have questions about adding therapeutic massage to your new and improved health care, ask your medical provider or mental health professional. Your employee wellness benefits may cover massage; scout out a local massage school for discounts.

The different types of massage include Swedish, deep tissue, sports massage, and trigger point, each focusing on a different way to provide healing and relaxation. Massage offers these important benefits, confirmed by ample research (Conrad 2022):

- Reduces stress

- Increases relaxation

- Reduces pain and muscle soreness and tension

- Improves circulation

- Increases energy and alertness

- Lowers heart rate and blood pressure

- Improves immune function

If any of these benefits speak to you, take a few moments to research a trusted professional in your area. Check out the American Massage Therapy Association to get started (https://www.amta massage.org/find-massage-therapist).

Other bodywork techniques—such as acupuncture, chiropractic, reiki, myofascial release, and shiatsu—can help you reconnect with your body and release stress. Choose a technique you know but haven't done in a long time, or a new one that you've wondered about.

● ● ● ● ●

Take a moment to answer these healing questions:

What can I offer my body today to be well?

What can I let go of in my body today to be well?

Engage with Your Body Checklist

Of the many ways you can engage with your body so it feels good and provides the strong foundation needed for your life without alcohol, choose one to focus on this week:

☐ Make one change to improve your sleep.

☐ Find a restorative yoga class online or in a local studio or gym, and try it.

☐ Add one more glass of water each day.

☐ Take a fifteen- to twenty-minute walk each day.

☐ Prioritize bodywork by setting aside money and scheduling an appointment with a licensed or certified bodywork practitioner.

Great! Now that you've listened to what your body needs to feel deeply well, let's explore ways to love your home and make it a healing sanctuary on your journey without alcohol. Get ready to welcome yourself home.

Chapter 3

Love Your Home

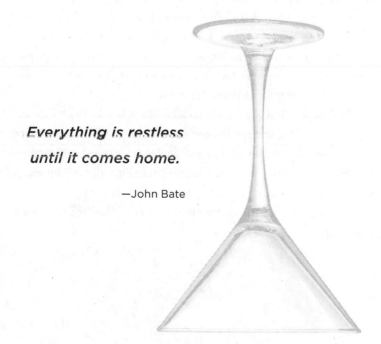

Everything is restless
until it comes home.

—John Bate

IF YOU'VE BEEN WAITING FOR THE RIGHT TIME to take care of your home, redecorate a room, move furniture around, repair a cabinet, organize a space, or get rid of unused or unloved objects, now could be a great time to tackle one of those projects. Whether you have roommates or a family or are single, rent your home or own it, your home is the *most important healing environment* in your alcohol-free life. Now that you're exploring a sober way of living, something special will be happening. You will be seeing your home in a different light—as a sanctuary from the stormy stressors of life.

How do you feel in your home right now? Are there places where you can pause and breathe? Do areas of your home make you smile and dance? Are you able to stay on top of your chores? Do you have a dedicated place to work and an inviting place to relax? This is a terrific opportunity to be kind and caring toward yourself and the haven of your home. When drinking is not the main focus, many people discover a bit of extra time (and even have a bit of extra money) to put toward a few small home improvements.

Let's explore healthy ways to reclaim your space and look forward to having your home warmly greet you each day. As you renegotiate your relationship to alcohol, you may find that you need new support from this sanctuary. I've chosen learning feng shui tips, decluttering with kindness, cleaning to music, making friends with your chores, and claiming your corner spot for healing. Let's fall in love with your home again.

11. Learn Feng Shui Tips

Feng shui is an ancient Chinese practice that uses energy forces to harmonize people with their surroundings. The term *feng shui* translates as "wind-water," and the idea is to mirror the flow of the natural environment within your home. A feng shui practitioner understands how landscapes and bodies of water impact *qi* or energy. Feng shui can help the practitioner understand the energy of your home and help improve the flow within it to increase wealth, happiness, health, and long life.

I am by no means a feng shui expert, but I have studied it and used the principles in my home and offices with great success. As I incorporated basic feng shui principles into my spaces, they just *felt* better. As a psychologist, clinic manager, and supervisor to students training to become mental health professionals, I've had thousands of staff members, clients, and students in my office spaces over more than twenty years. Many told me they felt incredibly relaxed in my office space and were able to express themselves freely and talk about difficult experiences. Some students have followed my lead and became more intentional about designing their office spaces as they invite in their own clients.

The principles of feng shui make perfect sense if you're embarking on a significant behavior change like discovering what it is like to be alcohol-free. Feng shui principles are intended to support you and your new goals in your home and work environments. Five natural elements—fire, water, metal, wood, and earth—set the stage for understanding this ancient practice. Each element has a related emotion: fear, anger, joy, sympathy, and grief, respectively (Benko

2016). Finding balance among these elements and learning ways to let emotions move through (without getting stuck or blocked) will help you feel grounded and calm.

Let's keep it simple and easy. Start with a few cleansing breaths and choose just one of these five areas of your home to focus on:

Front entrance. This space is an openhearted invitation for you, your family, and invited guests to arrive and feel good. Make sure your home's entrance is welcoming and uncluttered (look for another place for the family's shoes; store coats and bags in the closet). Replace your welcome mat with a fresh new one, and, if possible, add a plant or two on either side of the door.

Living room. Make sure there is enough room to comfortably move around the furniture. If the space feels crowded, you may need to remove one or two pieces. Minimize any sharp edges, and see if you can add more rounded lines in your art and cherished objects. Rounded edges allow the eyes to follow the lines more easily; they are less jarring and more similar to the lines found in nature.

Kitchen. Make sure this healing, nourishing space is clean and organized. Reduce clutter, receipts, paperwork, and toys on counters. Move items you use less frequently to a cabinet or pantry. Add inviting lighting and colorful plants when you get the chance. Showcase fresh fruit in a creative bowl as a simple daily reminder to focus on your health.

Bedroom. Perhaps the most soothing room in the home, it's your sanctuary at the end of a busy day when you need to offload disappointments, anxiety, and stress. Give your bedroom the respect it deserves. Make sure there is no unused furniture, idle workout equipment, dirty clothes, or kids' toys strewn about. If you can, ensure more restful sleep by removing electronics, including TV, computer, iPads, and cell phones. Artwork in greens and blues, similar to the green and blue spaces in nature, promotes well-being by reducing stress (Geneshka et al. 2021). And just like in nature, favor curved lines over straight edges in both furniture and objects.

Home office. If you're lucky enough to have a dedicated home office, that's terrific, but these simple tips also work for a small corner where you've set up a workspace. As in the other areas, your first step is clearing out any clutter and cleaning. File important papers in an organized, labeled bin and shred any papers you no longer need (check with a trusted online source to determine how long to keep important papers). Make sure the lighting is pleasing to your eyes and helpful for your work. Add a plant or fresh flowers to enhance the energy of the space.

The purpose here is to create space in your home and work settings that you love and that loves you back when you're making an important habit change like cutting down on alcohol. Of course, you don't need to tackle all of these areas at once. Take your time! First choose an area that may seem easy for you, then move on to more challenging areas. There is no rush; small changes can have a big impact. This is a lifelong process, with healing benefits that will be felt by you, others who live with you, and everyone you invite in.

12. Declutter with Kindness

This soothing strategy of *decluttering* is the kindest one in this chapter (and *all* the strategies are designed to be kind). There are plenty of decluttering tips, books, and podcasts out there for you to watch, read, or listen to. I encourage you to pick a favorite and follow along. Your home is now a place where you're *actively healing*. You may not realize that the extraneous items cluttering your home may have caused you anxiety and stress in the past. Some may even remind you of your drinking days. Now you're focusing on creating a home sanctuary to decrease anxiety, manage daily stress, and uplift your mood. It's an opportunity to gently reclaim your space and recharge your energy.

I'd like you to take on the decluttering experience with the idea that each space you give your decluttering attention to will serve to help you heal and make good decisions about not drinking.

I recommend starting with the kitchen—specifically, with the fridge, freezer, and pantry. Some recommend tackling a clothes closet, but the kitchen is a more neutral playing field, without the emotional connection to clothes, workout gear, bags, shoes, and jewelry. *Breathe.* Here we go.

Open your fridge and look at it with kindness. Remind yourself that it holds the sustenance for you and your family.

1. Take everything out.

2. Throw out any expired food and anything that no one plans to eat or drink.

3. Clean the inside and all storage parts with a good-smelling cleaner. Try a citrus scent; lemon enhances joy and positivity (Benko 2016).

4. Put back the fresh foods and beverages, organizing similar items together.

5. Make sure your refrigerator is set at the correct temperature.

6. If you have any alcohol in there, now's a good time to give it away or discard it (if the alcohol is your partner's or your roommates', see if you can put it in a designated place out of sight, so it's not the first thing you see whenever you open the fridge).

Great job! Next, let's move on to the freezer. Kindly acknowledge all the food it has been holding for you so that you have what you need to prepare meals far into the future.

7. Take everything out and throw away food that has been sitting there for too many weeks—or months.

8. Clean the inside with a good-smelling cleaner (again, try a citrus scent).

9. Make sure the freezer is set at the correct temperature.

10. Put back only food that you plan to eat within the next few months (check government food safety sites or *All Recipes* for guidelines on how long to store food safely and preserve freshness; some foods should not be frozen). Write the date on the package of the food to remind you to use it.

Wonderful! Now, let's tackle the pantry (or food storage cabinets). Thank the pantry for providing you the space to store food for yourself and your family.

11. Take everything out.

12. Throw away any expired food. (Take the trash out of the house as soon as you finish this project.)

13. Clean the shelves and walls with a good-smelling cleaner.

14. Put back all items in an organized way.

15. Make a shopping list for storage containers you may need to better organize your shelves for easy access.

16. When you get the containers, use them to organize in a pleasing way.

Nicely done. Let's keep going.

13. Clean with the Music On

My father worked for a time at Capitol Records in New York City, so we always had a diverse selection of music in our home. I experienced music as a way to connect our family, to be silly, dance, and have fun at home. The benefits of music to improve your well-being, enhance your mood, and decrease stress have been widely studied—and experienced by all of us. A wonderful, comprehensive research article by Dr. Daniel Gustavson and his colleagues (2021) of Vanderbilt University outlines the many benefits of music for supporting physical and mental health and decreasing substance use.

Many of the things we struggle with when newly sober can be helped by the following benefits of music:

- Lessening anxious feelings

- Improving depressive thoughts

- Managing post-traumatic stress symptoms

Let's here and now incorporate music into our daily chores. Choose music that's heartfelt; let the music connect with your mood.

Many years ago I worked in therapy with a couple who had two little kids and argued constantly about their mountain of chores: who would do them, who was doing more of them, and why the chores never seemed to end. Neither one thought about incorporating their favorite music into the tasks at hand. Their homework assignment was to each pick out ten favorite songs (that's over one hour of music) and use these songs to lighten the task of cleaning and tidying up around the house. When the music playlist was over, the family was allowed to stop the chores for the day.

This surprisingly easy assignment was a game changer for this family. Gone were the bad moods and resentment, and in their place was fun and lots of laughs as they danced and sang with their kids while attacking the daily chores.

Might it help to add a bit of musical joy to your daily chores? Here are a few suggested steps:

1. Start with music that you know and love or have loved in the past.

2. Find a playlist on your favorite music app that matches your mood for the tasks at hand (there are even playlists dedicated to cleaning!).

3. Use headphones if there are others in the house doing other activities. If you're alone, you can play your music all around your home.

4. If there are kids around, see if you can include some of their favorite songs and get everyone on board to tackle one chore—fold clean clothes, put clothes away, tidy up bedrooms, put toys away, put dishes in the dishwasher, put dishes away, vacuum, mop, dust, clean up the pet area, water the plants. You get the picture!

5. At the end of each day, choose three songs as a tidying-up playlist, and pick up items from the family room and kitchen. This way you will be greeted the next morning with a tidy home. Hurray!

Once you decide not to drink, you may have more time to devote to making your home more inviting for a quiet mind. Add your favorite music to the experience, and you're well on your way to creating a more healing environment. You can focus on musical ways to make tiny improvements to areas of your home that may have meant drudgery in the past. It's a fresh start, and it feels great.

14. Make Friends with Your Chores

I don't want you to be a perfectionist when it comes to your daily chores. We'll be taking a different approach to them now—one that is more mindful and less stressful. Even though, according to the Bureau of Labor Statistics, most of us in the U.S. devote about forty minutes per day to chores (that's almost five hours a week and over 240 hours per year!), they don't have to be the bane of your existence. If you don't have the budget for help with household tasks, not to worry. This is your opportunity to make friends with your chores as you fall in love with your home again. A clean, organized home will continue to assist, encourage, and enhance your sober journey. And we are officially going to put house cleaning and tidying in the category of exercise, so lots of extra benefit here. *Breathe.* Here are a few simple tips to make your five hours a week of chores enjoyable and successful:

- **Start with a vision.** Decide how you want your home to look. Take a few minutes to look online or in a magazine for a photo or two of an inspiration home. Then close your eyes, breathe, and imagine your home in a beautiful state of clean and calm.

- **Create an "I get to" list.** Write a short list of what you want to accomplish in this cleaning and tidying cycle, to help you stay on task. Remember, you're changing how you think, from *I have to* to *I get to* take great care of my home. You'll feel good as you get to check off your completed items.

- **Have a start time and, most important, an end time.**
  Don't make this an all-day event. Create a window of
  time when you do the work, and make sure you stop
  when you've reached the end point.

- **Change into your cleaning clothes.** Have a few pants
  and tops specifically for cleaning up. After your chores
  are done, take a shower or change into regular clothes
  to signal the end of the work.

- **Music (or an interesting podcast) makes everything
  better.** Tip #13 bears repeating here. Ask friends what
  music or podcast they like to listen to while cleaning, and
  see if you can expand your cleaning horizon.

- **Design your own cleaning products.** You can create
  wonderful cleaning supplies to make your home smell
  and feel good all day. Test essential oils that make you
  feel happy, and design your signature home scent.

When you're taking care of your home, slow down and change
how you think about the experience. Focus on the task at hand. These
tasks will feel different now that you're taking a break from alcohol,
because you will be better able to focus without feeling resentful or
distracted. When you're doing the laundry, focus on doing the
laundry. When you're doing the dishes, focus on doing the dishes.
Release any judgment. Be kind to the part of you that loves and cares
for your home. Your home is your and your family's safe place and
sanctuary from the busy, stressful world outside. As alcohol becomes
less important in your life, you might be surprised to start looking
forward to taking care of your space and creating a healing environment—your soft place to land.

15. Claim Your Corner Spot

Having a small space you can call your own is possibly one of the most important pieces of your healing puzzle. Deciding what spot to claim as yours is not something to brush off or put off to another day. Today is the day. *Breathe* and follow these simple steps:

1. Take a look around your home and determine where you can set up a space to meditate, read, think, or just be.

2. Be creative with your choice; see if you can make it a place that you look forward to returning to day after day. If you're lucky enough to live in a warmer climate, you may want to choose a little outdoor nook for yourself.

3. Set up your newfound space with a few treasured items, a pillow or blanket to sit on, perhaps a candle, a journal and a cherished pen, and an inspirational or meditation book. One of my favorites is Melody Beattie's *Journey to the Heart: Daily Meditations on the Path to Freeing Your Soul* or, if you want to focus a bit more on sobriety, try our book *The Gift of Recovery: 52 Ways to Live Joyfully Beyond Addiction* by Rebecca Williams and Julie Kraft.

4. Bring a cup of tea to your beloved area. Sip and reflect on how you'd like this space to take care of you and help you start your day or return from an especially difficult day.

5. Make it a no-media zone. Do not do work here. Please don't answer your emails, text, or scroll here. It's just a

small space to unplug from the world for ten minutes each day.

6. Chances are, once you establish your space, kids and pets will want to join you. This is normal, since they will notice the positive, calm energy of your space. Kids and pets are welcome. Show your kids, cats, and dogs that this is a quiet space. Teach your kids how to have a few minutes of resting, writing, drawing, doing nothing, or napping. Give your pets a corner to rest in too. Once they see you're quiet, they will follow suit.

The goal is to return to this space once or twice each day, usually first thing in the morning and last thing at night. It may also be useful as a boundary time between work life and home life. Don't force it. Your corner spot is waiting for you. Make it a welcoming sanctuary.

● ● ● ● ●

Each day, take a moment to answer these healing questions:

What can I offer my home sanctuary today?

What can I let go of in my home sanctuary today?

Love Your Home Checklist

How will you know when you've been able to love your home so that your home welcomes you and supports your life without alcohol? Which of the following suggestions could you can take action on? Choose one to focus on this week:

- ☐ Learn about feng shui to support yourself and your home as you make lifestyle changes.

- ☐ Begin the "decluttering with kindness" experience. Choose just one room of your home to start with.

- ☐ Create a music play list and listen to it during your daily chores.

- ☐ Choose to make friends with one of your chores.

- ☐ Designate and arrange a corner spot just for you. Place inspirational objects or a treasured book there. Sip your favorite tea in your new space.

Terrific! Now it's time to venture into the natural environment to continue to explore balance and expand your well-being. Let's see what you discover.

Chapter 4

Rediscover Nature

I firmly believe that nature brings solace to all troubles.

—Anne Frank

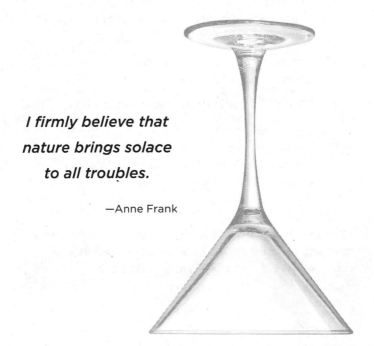

MANY OF US HAVE BEEN GIVEN the mistaken message that we do not have a green thumb. Mention houseplants, and we shrink like a violet. When I was growing up in a small apartment in the Bronx, no one in my neighborhood had indoor plants, and it was next to impossible to find plants sold in the local stores. The urban landscape was a scene of concrete, brick, and tall buildings blocking out the sun and sky.

My family did go to the New York Botanical Gardens regularly. It was my mother's favorite place in all of New York City. I didn't know then how important indoor plants, outdoor gardens, and wildlife would become to me.

Now I always gravitate to having plants in my home, and whatever new community I find myself in, I make every effort to go out exploring green areas. If I haven't had a chance to get my nature fix outside, I tend to gravitate to watching nature documentaries. It's the next best thing.

Think for a moment about how you grew up. Did you have plants around? Did you go out into nature regularly? If you did, but you haven't focused on your natural environment for a while, this is a great opportunity to reintroduce green into your life and rediscover nature and feel how it expands your mood.

Inviting nature and plants into your life, now that you're trying on an alcohol-free lifestyle, is a powerful way to slow down, get grounded, and reconnect with yourself. Your new reality can be summed up in the following phrases: *I have a green thumb, I love being out in nature, I find creative ways to bring nature into my home*. If you've bought into the *I don't have a green thumb* judgment, your ability to nurture indoor plants may surprise you. You're going to love being out in nature or just being outside. These positive thoughts will trigger a change in you.

Your connection with the natural world is always there for you to come back to and enjoy. It's especially helpful to return to nature when you're feeling overwhelmed, when you have cravings for alcohol, or when you're questioning your decision to not drink. It's good to know there is research supporting the fact that being in nature can decrease the strength and frequency of addiction cravings (Martin et al. 2019).

Let's start with creating and enjoying your indoor sanctuary, then get outside to explore your outdoor oasis. You'll seek out opportunities to immerse yourself in nature, find your creative spark and draw or write while outside, or even watch a nature documentary to embrace this new type of healing. Ready to rediscover nature?

16. Cultivate Your Indoor Sanctuary

As you learn how to live joyfully without alcohol, having a small indoor green space will greatly benefit your mood. Here, smaller is better. Start with just one or two indoor potted plants, ones that are easy to grow inside. I tend to rescue potted plants from my local grocery store, but feel free to take a trip to a nursery or home improvement store if you have one nearby. Ask friends and family if there are any plants they no longer want to care for, and offer to take them off their hands. Hint that you'd like an indoor plant as a gift for an upcoming birthday or holiday. Sometimes you can find inexpensive plants at farmers' markets or local flea markets. Even going to a yard sale or moving sale is a creative way to score mature houseplants at little to no cost. (Check out *The Spruce* online for even more inspiration for finding and nurturing your new plants.)

Once you have your new plant babies, follow these simple steps:

1. Create a few spaces close to the windows for your plants to enjoy their new home and lap up a bit of sunshine.

2. Follow the sunlight, watering, and fertilizing instructions on the tag that comes with the plant.

3. Even better, look up the name of the plant you've purchased and research its particular needs. Many of us tend to overwater—I like to call it *overlove*—our houseplants, thinking we're doing them a favor. Most plants need

time to absorb the water you give them and dry out a bit before you give them more.

4. Talk to your plants, listen to your plants, rotate them to get light on all sides, and enjoy what they give you each day. Your plants will clean your indoor air and give your mood a boost. They can even give you a bit of privacy from your neighbors or between your interior spaces.

Something special happens when you're experiencing sobriety and spending time caring for your plants. This care is emblematic of how you're caring for and nurturing yourself. As you watch your plants flourish, also notice yourself flourishing. Without drinking, you have more focus and attention to give to yourself and your plants. It's a win-win.

If you can't afford to buy a bunch of books on plants right now, check your local library. Read blogs by houseplant experts to get a handle on your houseplant journey. Be sure to put a plant in your new corner spot or your home office area to activate positive energy. Expect yourself and your home to start to feel better—and you just might develop a new plant hobby!

17. Enjoy Your Outdoor Oasis

From cultivating your small (but mighty) indoor garden, we move on to discovering your outdoor oasis. Even if you don't have a big garden or green space outside, all you need is a window box, a patio, or a deck with a bit of space to experience the amazing benefits of outdoor plants.

When you're outside, feel the energy of the green space: grass, bushes, flowers, and trees. Notice anything that is blooming or has completed a bloom cycle. What season is it right now? Notice how your outdoor areas change with the seasons. Study the plants native to your region and choose ones that are hardy for your environment. Get your hands in the dirt to plant flowers or other greenery. Take a moment to smell the soil, the fertilizer, and the plants. Notice how you feel.

If you don't have any outdoor greenery of your own, explore your neighborhood for well-known or hidden green spaces and try one of these tips:

- Take a walk and look at your local plants and trees with fresh eyes. Mindfully, notice the different shades of green and any new flowers that are blooming.

- If you're in the middle of the city, scout out a local park or a tree-lined street. Slow down and wander.

- Find a bench to sit on and enjoy the trees and listen to the birds. Take note of how many different bird songs you hear.

- If you're walking, take a moment to look around, look up, and enjoy the majesty of an entire tree. Estimate how tall the tree is; think about how old the tree is.

- *Breathe.* Enjoy the fresh air. Take long, deep, slow breaths and appreciate the natural world at your doorstep.

Spending time outdoors has been shown to have a positive effect on regulating our mood and our thinking. Being outside among the trees helps decrease the fight-or-flight hormones like adrenaline and cortisol that course through our bodies when we're stressed. These hormones might be out of balance when you first stop drinking alcohol. As you relax and renew outside, your body increases serotonin endorphins—the feel-good neurotransmitters that have a calming effect on your overall mood and mental health. An added benefit you might notice from being outside (and taking short breaks from your phone) is an improvement in your attention and focus. Great reasons to carve out time to get outside. The rewards are priceless.

18. Explore Nature Trails

Now let's venture farther into nature. Being in nature has wonderful effects on your mood. If you're having challenges with anxiety or depression as you begin to remove alcohol from your days, nature is there to help. Getting outside will increase your oxygen intake and decrease your cortisol levels, both of which decrease stress and help you relax your mind and breathe easier. Being in nature also gives you the space to consider why you were drinking and what the drinking may have been covering up. Getting some clarity is always a good thing.

Look up nature trails or hiking trails in your area. We don't all have a nature trail in our backyard or have access to a nature trail at all. Be creative. Sometimes nature trails can be found in wildlife refuges, botanical gardens, or even local zoos. Research has shown the importance of nature in recovery from mental health challenges and substance use, as it decreases stress and increases well-being (Martin et al. 2020; Bratman, Olvera-Alvarez, and Gross 2021). You owe it to yourself and your overall health to get outside and explore your natural environment. This is also a great opportunity to invite a friend along with you or take your family on a new adventure. *Breathe*.

Ask your local community groups to recommend nature walks. There may be some hidden gems, new to you and perfect for that nature getaway. If you're lucky enough to live near a coast, get to the beach with your friends or family. Explore new and less popular areas and start a list of places you'd like to return to.

Make greenery—whether in your home or outside—part of your new healing journey. Notice the small moments of improved mood, better coping, and overall slowing down. As you move through life with a renewed focus on nature, you can continue shifting your thinking about alcohol's role in your life.

19. Write or Draw for Growth

As you're experiencing nature and watching your indoor plants grow, it might be a good time to incorporate art and creativity into your life. The natural environment is one of the best places to find inspiration. Even a small patch of green or a neighborhood park may spark ideas. Sometimes reading about nature is a great starting point; for instance, in Mary Oliver's poetry collection *Devotion* (2020), many of the poems are about the natural world, interacting with it and being a part of it. Read a poem out loud, and see what comes up for you.

Check your local library for gardening and nature books and magazines. Sometimes reading about the natural world or looking at beautiful nature photographs can trigger a burst of creativity. Writing or drawing can also help you feel grounded in nature. Here are a few ideas and prompts to get the nature energy flowing, whether by writing or drawing:

Writing

1. Bring a notebook or journal and favorite pen to a local green area.

2. Find a bench or other comfortable place to sit, then open your journal and explore, uncover, and create.

3. *Breathe.* Begin writing by describing what you see. Trees, flowers, shrubs, dogs strolling by, the clouds forming shapes in the sky, kids wandering around. Describe the weather and signs of the season and how you respond to these.

4. Use the following prompts to forge a deeper connection to where you are. Write a paragraph each for only four of these prompts. Spend twenty minutes writing (about five minutes per prompt). Remember to release all judgment. If any critical thoughts come into your mind, let them float away like the clouds moving through the sky.

● This area reminds me of a time when…

● I love being in nature with my…

● I feel connected to the trees because…

● When my mind quiets down, I am able to…

● I am grateful for the way…

● When I look up, I see…

● I feel relaxed here because…

● My heart is leading me to…

Drawing

1. Bring drawing paper and colored pens or pencils to a local green area.

2. Find a bench or other comfortable place to sit.

3. *Breathe.* Look around and take in the beauty of the plants and trees.

4. Pick a tree to sketch and begin. Remember to release all judgment; enjoy that creative freedom that young children feel when drawing.

5. Spend twenty minutes drawing.

Nature can help you when you're overwhelmed and craving alcohol. Being outside can also help your mood and your ability to reclaim your calm. One way to harness nature's calming ability and decrease any cravings you may have is to channel it into creative outlets. If you'd like to take this experience to the next level, see if you can find a local art or writing class that focuses on natural surroundings.

20. Watch Your Nature

If you've had a long week at work, are unable to get outside at all, or are just too exhausted, there is another way to get your nature fix. There are lots of excellent nature documentaries available that can soothe your mind and make you feel like you're actually in nature. And research backs up the idea that watching nature can be just as good as being outside in it. You can feel connected to nature and experience that sense of well-being by watching nature documentaries (Martin et al. 2020; Young-Mason 2020). These studies also indicate this helps ease fear and anxiety and nurtures a deeper appreciation for the natural world.

To fall in love with watching your nature, try these tips:

- Google the best (or the top ten) nature documentaries and choose one that piques your interest, or ask your family which one they'd like to watch.

- Plan an evening and give yourself about ninety minutes of uninterrupted time to dive into a documentary.

- Make it a legitimate movie night with popcorn and your favorite nonalcoholic beverages.

- Be in the moment and imagine yourself in the movie— or directing it.

- Feel your mind slow down, and enjoy your connection with nature.

- If this is something that you love, why not plan for another nature night?

When you're in the mood to look at nature with music and no narration, try *Moving Art* on Netflix. Keep in mind that each of us experiences connection to nature in our own unique way. What nature documentary works for you may not resonate with your family members, and vice versa. You're just gathering information here. There are no hard and fast rules.

Sometimes listening to nature sounds at home—like rain, or the ocean, or the forest—works best. You can even play nature music when you're enjoying your daily meditation; give yourself fifteen minutes and notice how you feel. What a brilliant and easy way to unwind!

Ask yourself these healing questions:

What can I offer myself to rediscover nature today?

What can I let go of in order to rediscover nature today?

Rediscover Nature Checklist

How will you know when you've been able to rediscover your indoor and outdoor garden or natural environment? Look at the checklist items and see which tip speaks to you. Choose one area to focus on this week:

- ☐ Add a plant or two to create an indoor sanctuary where you can unwind and relax.

- ☐ Create an outdoor oasis or visit a local oasis to help with your mood and give you room to breathe.

- ☐ Explore nature trails or outdoor green spaces to heal and destress.

- ☐ Uncover ways to write or draw to reconnect with nature and reaffirm your decision to take a break from drinking.

- ☐ Choose one nature documentary to watch, or spend fifteen minutes listening to nature sounds.

Wonderful! Now that you've discovered your surprising green thumb, explored the healing green spaces around you, or enjoyed nature documentaries in your home, it's time to venture out and give some love to your relationships. This is getting interesting!

Chapter 5

Nurture Your Relationships

Your heart is the
softest place on
earth. Take care of it.

—Nayyirah Waheed

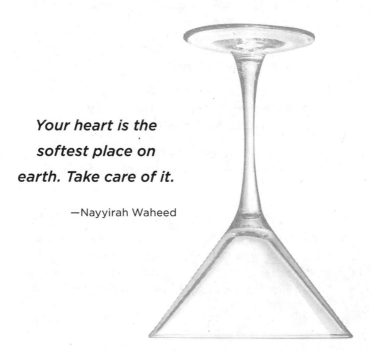

IT'S TRULY SHOCKING HOW YOUR RELATIONSHIPS change as you give up alcohol and step into a sober lifestyle. Someone you first thought was a dyed-in-the-wool best friend now is someone you don't talk to at all. Some folks that you had a good relationship with may have fallen away completely. You may wonder whether the rift is your fault, racking your brain to try to figure out what you did "wrong" to have caused these breakups. Or you may be surprised that people you used to hang out with have absolutely no appeal to you anymore, and you find yourself making excuses to *not* see them.

You're healing and changing every day, so give yourself some slack and be patient as you move through this uncharted territory in your life. It may be time to heal old friendships and explore new connections.

Making friends is never easy, but you may find yourself gravitating to others who have the same interests as you or who also have decided to be alcohol-free. You may rekindle old friendships that fell away years ago. Essentially, everyone—and I mean *everyone*—goes through relationship changes when they decide to stop drinking alcohol. You're definitely not alone, even if you feel alone at the moment. Perhaps a few of these soothing techniques will help you take care of the relationships you wish to nurture and build new relationships that support where you are now. Let's embrace new communication skills, figure out ways to renegotiate your relationships for healing, schedule down time to recharge, learn simple ways to rebuild old and new friendships, and explore imaginative ways to have fun. As always, proceed slowly and be kind to yourself.

21. Embrace New Communication Skills

If you're finding it difficult to communicate with others now that you're not relying on drinking, know that this is very common. Are others finding it difficult (or awkward) to communicate with you? Also very common. Without alcohol on board, all that *social anxiety* that you might have been masking with it might just flood back into your interactions with others.

Let's figure out together a few new communication skills that can get you through the rough patches. I don't want you to force things—there's no need to make it hard on yourself right now. Try out these skills and see if they fit. And if they don't fit, give something else a try. Be flexible here.

The first skill, and possibly the hardest at the beginning of not drinking, is to *be honest* with the people in your life. But before you can be honest with others, it makes sense to make sure you're being honest with yourself. This means saying the truth about what is going on with you. It's being open and clear about where you are in your life and about your decision to not drink alcohol. When you're talking to yourself, it may sound something like this:

Today I am choosing to not drink alcohol.

This decision is in my best interest, and I like who I am when I don't drink.

My mind is much clearer when I choose not to drink; I like this feeling.

I'm beginning to feel healthier without alcohol, so I'm going to continue on this path.

The second skill, when you're talking to other people who may not understand what you're doing or interacting with people you used to drink with, is to *offer open questions.* Open questions don't allow for a yes or no response; they provide space for exploration. Make sure you choose an appropriate time and place when broaching the subject. The questions may sound something like the following (choose one question to start):

Is now a good time to talk about what has been going on with us?

I'm healing day to day; what things feel different with us since I've decided to stop drinking?

I know our relationship is changing; what have you noticed?

Thanks for being open-minded. What changes do you like and what changes don't you like?

After you ask a question, leave space open to see where the conversation goes. Listen without judgment of yourself or the other person. There are no right answers to these questions. Each relationship is unique. As you reflect on how this relationship has been in the past, chances are you'll feel like things are shifting. Accept how it is now; try not to slip into negativity or blaming. Be kind to yourself. Don't force it. And if possible, show some kindness toward the other person, even if you disagree.

The third skill is to *express empathy*—the ability to see things from the other person's perspective. You're developing your empathy muscle (which may have atrophied when you were drinking alcohol and not experiencing your true feelings). Here are some helpful phrases for talking to a friend about your choice to cut down or stop drinking:

> *I bet this has been difficult for you.*

> *I get that you're feeling hurt, alone, and disregarded.*

> *Let's see if we can work through this together.*

> *I imagine you're worried our relationship feels different, and you want the old me back.*

See if you and your friend together can come up with one or two ways to give respect to the problem. For instance, you can say "How about if we talk once a week and give some time to exploring how our relationship is changing? Let's make sure we talk about the challenges *and* the good things that are happening for both of us."

Remember, you're practicing new communication skills, and you won't master them all at once. As you practice honest communication, active listening, and empathy skills, it may be one step forward and two steps back. If an interaction goes south or really agitates you, use one of the other ways to unwind offered in this book. Not everyone is going to understand your choices, especially if they knew you only as someone they've had drinks with over the years. Cultivating these new communications skills will be worth it in the long run, so stick with it for those people you truly care about and want in your life.

22. Renegotiate for Healing

Once you've practiced a few simple ways to communicate with one or two people in your circle of friends, it's time to renegotiate what you need for your personal healing. This usually includes understanding your boundaries when it comes to your relationships. Part of being honest with yourself and with others is to figure out *your* specific boundaries.

Relationship boundaries allow us to embrace the differences between us and our friends in a healthy, respectful way. Now that you're not drinking, it may be a good time talk about what you need in the relationship and to hear what your friend needs. For example, if you've decided to not go out to bars on the weekends, what other activities can you do with your friends that will be mutually enjoyable and a good way to destress? Here is an example of how to renegotiate your relationship for healing:

> *Our friendship is important to me.*
>
> *Now that I've decided not to drink, I wonder if we can do other activities together to reconnect and have fun.*
>
> *I have a few ideas; what are some things you would like to do?*

People in your life will not automatically know when they've crossed one of your boundaries. If you feel angry, disappointed, burned out, exhausted, or puzzled, it's likely a boundary has been crossed. If these feelings hang around a bit too long and you can't shake them, it may be time to reflect on how you can broach the boundary subject. It's usually better not to wait too long to talk about your boundaries. *Breathe*. There will be growing pains as you recalibrate yourself and your relationships without drinking. Keep in mind that some relationships may not survive the leap from the drinking you to the not-drinking you. Making changes can be challenging, but it is part of your well-being and growth as a human being. Those who have your best interests at heart are the ones you need most during this time. And these relationships are the ones you can offer the most to as you grow and change.

23. Schedule Your Down Time

It's important to actually schedule some down time *every day*. This is time for you to recharge so that you have more to give to yourself and others. Let's face it, well-meaning people (even people you really love) can drain your precious energy and leave you feeling spent. And I do mean schedule it in your calendar or on your to-do list. Here are some suggestions:

- Meditate for fifteen minutes.

- Take a nap.

- Read your favorite book.

- Listen to your favorite podcast or playlist.

- Repot plants.

- Sit on a bench, daydream and enjoy the view.

- Cuddle up with a blanket in your cozy chair.

- Spend time with your pets.

The goal is to acquire more internal resources for when you go back out to meet your friends, spend time with your family, or reengage in the workplace. Over time, these small moments will definitely make a big difference to your mood and functioning. Because you're not drinking, chances are you will notice others' needs more acutely now. You may need to deflect bad jokes, block judgments, and sidestep drama in ways you didn't have to in the past. You might notice that you're feeling everything more intensely now without alcohol to numb you or take the edge off. So make sure you give your mind a chance to heal. Proceed gradually.

I'm a big fan of preparing hours or days in advance for any upcoming event with lots of folks or even a small group of two or three. It's also essential that you not judge yourself when you take some time to revitalize yourself. It is not selfish to focus on yourself. Calling yourself selfish is a false narrative, not fact. Sometimes these negative thoughts are a sign that you're feeling burned out. To prevent yourself from becoming more burned out, change how you narrate your story. Change the word from *self-ish* to *self-healing* or *self-love*. Scheduling down time is about soothing yourself, and you're worth the extra time to recharge the batteries and reset for the world outside.

24. Rebuild Old and New Friendships

Once you've decided that a friendship can withstand a big change like quitting drinking, it's time to rebuild. And it's possible you can rebuild a stronger, more satisfying friendship now that you've gotten past the rough patches.

This is where honest communication comes into play. Be clear and kind about where you are in your life, how you're making choices, and what is important to you. *Try to not offer advice to your friends about their drinking behavior unless they specifically ask for it.* Everyone is on their own journey. Talk about what is working well for you, how you're feeling a bit healthier, and how you're navigating your new feelings and behaviors.

Along with building old friendships, there is the daunting task of developing new friendships. If this makes you want to run for the hills, you're not alone. Most people who have made a major behavior change, like you have, will experience growing pains when it comes to anything new. You may now feel shy and awkward—feelings that you may have covered up with alcohol in the past. Keep in mind that your feelings are normal as you learn new ways to relate with others. Sometimes it's helpful to meet other people who have decided not to drink or to meet up with a group of people who are taking a break from alcohol or trying the sober lifestyle, to practice socializing. *Breathe.* Acknowledge that you're feeling uncomfortable and vulnerable with your new friends. Chances are they are feeling the same way.

As you learn new ways to navigate new friendships, it's important to follow up and let the other person know that you enjoyed the time together. If you like the person and, more important, like who you are with the person, plan another time together and keep the positive relationship energy flowing. Give yourself some slack: Doing anything new requires a period of adjustment, and this is certainly no different.

If you've lost a friendship, give yourself time and space to heal. Try your very best not to speak badly about the other person—and offer a loving-kindness prayer to yourself and the other person. Offering kindness—both to yourself and to others—is a wonderful and powerful way to be mindful (developed by Sharon Salzberg, 2018) and to respect the changes you're making. Here is an example of a loving-kindness prayer you might like to write in your journal, copy onto your phone, and say out loud to see how it feels:

May I be safe.

May I be happy.

May I be healthy.

May I live with ease.

Once you've offered this loving-kindness meditation to yourself, try the next step, offering it to your lost friend:

May my friend be safe.

May my friend be happy.

May my friend be healthy.

May my friend live with ease.

Repeat these phrases a few times each day as you begin to calm your central nervous system and offer yourself the kindness you deserve as you grieve the loss of a friendship. You're going to make it through this difficult passage. Be patient; it will take some time.

25. Explore New Ways to Have Fun

Sometimes when you stop drinking alcohol or stop doing activities that center around alcohol, it may feel like you'll never have fun again. Thoughts like these might pop into your mind:

People will think I'm a total bore.

No one will invite me to their parties.

I don't know what to do with myself when I do go out.

I don't know how to interact with other people.

I feel stiff and uptight.

Why do I want to turn around and leave social situations?

It's true, you will be going through a period of transition. You will be evolving from a person who interacts with others while drinking to a person who interacts with others without drinking. There might be lots of fish-out-of-water moments and confusing interactions. This transition may feel like it's going on forever. *Breathe.* It also brings lots of opportunities to learn about yourself and determine who you are, who you'd like to hang out with, and where you want to spend your precious time.

Now that you've decided to not have alcohol as a primary player in your life, you will most likely need to make a few friends or acquaintances who do not drink. Research alcohol-free events or sober book clubs in your area. These folks will understand what you're going through and lend a sympathetic ear as you navigate your decisions. Be sure to stock up on cool alcohol-free mocktails at home to serve your new friends (check out chapter 7, tip 35, for more ideas).

It's important to explore creative ways to bring excitement into your alcohol-free lifestyle. As you explore new ways to turn up the fun, keep your commitment to not drinking as a top priority. Think about what you used to do for fun *before* you started drinking at every event, and answer these questions:

- What captured your interest?

- What hobby, activity, or group of people did you keep coming back to again and again?

- What put a smile on your face?

- When did you feel most playful?

- When was the last time you had a real belly laugh?

Look at a photograph of yourself as a smiley, happy little kid. What positive feelings do you have when you look at your younger self? She looks like a blast! He's so curious. She likes to solve puzzles. He's really funny. These are the places we want to explore again. There may be enjoyable activities that have never crossed your mind before. Now is a good time to make a list of possible fun activities that you'd like to try with a sober friend. Choose one of these small activities to share over the next week:

- Try a new recipe.

- Rearrange the furniture in your living room.

- Go out to a movie.

- Have brunch at an up-and-coming restaurant.

- Take a painting class.

- Go to a local bookstore.

- Watch sports together.

- Visit a botanical garden.

- Go for a walk around your neighborhood.

- Listen to live music in your community.

Don't overthink it; keep things doable. It may take a few tries to find the activity that speaks to you and your friend.

If you and your friend have kids close to the same age, explore activities for your families that bring out the kid in all of you. Choose one of these or think up one of your own:

- Plan a trip to the zoo or aquarium (this can be virtual or in person).

- Take a walk and look for wildlife.

- Visit a local beach or lake.

- Go on a bike ride.

- Do puzzles or play cards together.

- Have a baking party.

- Learn how to garden.

- Visit your local library.

- Go to a sports event.

There is no limit to the possibilities you can pursue now that your mind is clear and you're inviting new experiences into your life (or revisiting some favorites). Remember, you're practicing new friendship skills, so take it slow and easy. You're headed in a great direction.

● ● ● ● ●

Take a moment to honestly answer these healing questions:

What can I offer one of my relationships today?

What can I let go of in one of my relationships today?

Nurture Your Relationships Checklist

How will you know when you've been able to nurture your relationships so that they feel strong, vibrant, and supportive without alcohol in the mix? Take a look at these relationship areas and choose one to focus your energy on this week:

- ☐ Choose one communication skill to try this week: Be honest, ask open questions, or show empathy.

- ☐ Give yourself time to renegotiate one of your relationships so that both parties have a sense of support and healing.

- ☐ Schedule down time this week so you can recharge your batteries and revive your internal resources.

- ☐ Choose one activity for rebuilding a friendship or developing a new friendship.

- ☐ Begin to design a life without drinking that includes one creative way to have fun this week.

Navigating relationships as you begin to move through life with less alcohol or no alcohol is not always easy, but the rewards are waiting for you. Next, we are going to consider how you can reconnect with your work, where you spend lots of time each day.

Chapter 6

Reconnect with Your Work

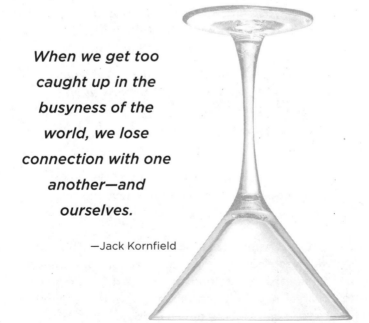

When we get too caught up in the busyness of the world, we lose connection with one another—and ourselves.

—Jack Kornfield

WORK HAS CHANGED QUITE A BIT from the old traditional ways for almost everyone. People are making decisions about how, where, and how much they want to work like never before. As you begin to change your relationship with alcohol, you may be feeling differently about how you spend most of each work day too. You may have new clarity about what type of work you do, who you'd like to work with, and how much time you want to spend working. You may have been able to move your work from the office setting to your home. Or you may be starting a job in an exciting or challenging new environment.

Let's tackle a few skills that could help you stay healthy as you make these important changes and reconnect with work. Understanding the importance of work life boundaries, making your home work for you, reclaiming your work friends, respecting your desk (wherever it is), and cultivating the characteristics of a great boss are all ways you can deeply realign with your work. Some of these tips might be just the ticket to a healthier working life.

26. Build Boundaries for Wellness

Creating boundaries at work could be important to your well-being. If you're commonly feeling overextended and undervalued, that may lead you to use alcohol as a way to cope. Having a clear set of guidelines to help you separate your work life from your nonwork life may be one of your best coping strategies. It's a way to give yourself a break from the demands of work and reclaim space to breathe. Whether you've been at the same job for years or you're starting something new, it's in your best interest to set some boundaries. To feel better when you work, try one of these suggestions.

Assess Your Inner Resources

How are you feeling when you get to work, and throughout your workday? Are you angry, stressed, or resentful? As you begin to construct healthy boundaries, you'll want to build up a supply of inner resources to tap into if you have a rough day or week. This means taking breaks in your day, taking time off, getting support from a work colleague, or getting professional support.

Practice Stating What You Can and Cannot Do

It can feel daunting to speak up clearly, whether in person or in an email, about what is possible (or not possible) for you to tackle in your day or on a project. That's why I recommend you practice a few key phrases that are calm and clear about your time limits and your ability to complete a project. *Breathe.* I call these phrases "positive sandwiches:" You start with a positive connection, state clearly in the middle that you're not able to do the work requested, and end with another positive connection. As you practice this skill, try sandwiches like these:

"Thank you for considering me for this assignment. Due to my current workload, I will not be able to take it on right now. Please think of me for other upcoming assignments."

"This new project sounds interesting. When I complete what I am working on, I will definitely give it consideration. Thanks for thinking of me for this project."

Follow Up with a Calm Mind

Another important way to take care of yourself is to give yourself time to review what you're being asked to do. See if a response like "Let me review what you're requesting, and I'll let you know if I am available to meet your needs" makes sense for you to get a little breathing room. Let the other person or your boss know when you will get back to them (an hour, a day, or a week), and stick to your word. Of course, as you use these boundary-clarifying phrases you might get pushback. This is normal; being kind but firm is the best way to take care of yourself and your well-being. When someone has asked you to complete a project, don't just leave them hanging. To help protect your boundaries, make sure you follow up with the person who made the request. Then when your schedule frees up a bit, let them know.

The goal here is to establish and maintain good healthy relationships with everyone who works with you.

27. Make Your Home Work for Work

Let's face it: Working from home has a big upside. Less commuting on public transportation, fewer cars on the road, less wear and tear on your car, less rushing to get to work on time, and less face-to-face interacting when you just don't feel like it. The humorous (but often true) phrase "This meeting could have been an email" comes into sharp focus when you begin to account for the time spent.

But there is big downside too. Many who work from home report working longer hours, feeling disconnected from their colleagues, and experiencing more loneliness and depressed mood. So you might need to make some small changes to how you work from home to make it work a little better for you.

On the plus side, since changing your drinking habits, you might enjoy time at home to regroup and rebuild yourself.

How you feel about working from home may depend on whether you're more of an introvert or an extrovert. Here are a few keys to setting yourself up for success if you'll be working from home, either part-time or full-time. Choose one or two—and fall in love with working from home:

Set yourself up. One way that may help you get into the work mentality at home is to dress the part: Shower and dress as if you are going to the office. (Do be comfortable.) This signals your mind that you're transitioning to work and ready for anything that the workday might bring your way. You might also benefit from relying on regular rituals like a to-do list, maintaining your hours on a timesheet, or ensuring a tidy, welcoming workspace.

Set up your space. Having a space in your home that is conducive to productivity is the holy grail of working from home. You need quiet in order to focus. If you're lucky enough to have a dedicated office space with a door, fantastic. If not, create the space that makes the most sense for you and your work needs. Make sure you have your office supplies handy. Keep things simple, private, and uncluttered.

Set up your time. You'll need to decide when your work hours begin and end. Try to stay within the bounds you set for your work schedule, whether it's full-time, like a 9-to-5 day, or part-time, like a 10-to-2 day. You might set your phone alarm to alert you to the end of your workday. To maintain separation between your work and personal lives, try to not respond to work emails or texts after hours, unless you're on call or there's an emergency. Tidy up your desk, and leave your work space ready for the next work day.

Set up your breaks. You do not want to sit at your desk for hours at a stretch, until you're so stiff you can barely get up. It's your responsibility to take care of yourself. At regular intervals, get up, stretch, walk around, go outside, breathe deeply, or even lie down for a few minutes. Look for a break reminder program you can set up on your system. There are online yoga classes designed to be done in the middle of a workday if you're stuck at your desk. To prevent eye strain, take breaks to look away from the computer monitor. Follow the 20-20-20 rule recommended by the Mayo Clinic (2022) for optimum eye health: Every twenty minutes, look at something twenty feet away for at least twenty seconds.

Set up your goals. Working in this new work environment requires us to be realistic about how much we can get done in any given day or week. Having achievable goals is important for your mental and emotional well-being, especially for those new to working from home. Get down to business by writing down what you want to accomplish, and communicate with your boss and coworkers about your plans to tackle the work at hand. Take breaks between projects, and celebrate all of your achievements, big and small.

Set up your computer. Technology is going to be your best friend now that you're working from home. Invest in a computer that will make your home work life as easy as possible. Make sure you have the best internet connection available, and download the apps you'll need to support your work. You may need to talk to your employer about the necessary equipment. This all requires upfront money; see if your employer offers resources.

Set up your kid, pets, partner, roommates, parents, and houseguests. Is your home full of people and pets? That's pretty common. Make sure your kids have something educational or fun to do while you're working. Most likely, you will need to take short breaks to check on them. Check in with your partner to let them know you've designated specific time to work; you'll catch up with them on one of your breaks, at lunchtime, or at dinner. Decide whether to allow your pets into your workspace (chances are your furry friends will want to be in on the action), and give them a bed nearby. Give houseguests ideas for exploring the town while you're working. Plan to meet up with them at dinner time. Also, plan to meet up with your roommate at the end of the work day to catch up.

Set up your food and beverage. One tricky thing that happens when you work from home is *food creep*. Somehow snacks magically appear on your desk, sometimes multiple times each day. Your kitchen and pantry are steps away; it can be difficult to ignore how close all your food is now. Set some guidelines for eating. Schedule lunch, and embrace the time you have for it. And give yourself guidelines on snacks too. As for beverages, treat yourself well: Splurge on good coffee, calming tea, hot chocolate, or inventive nonalcoholic cold drinks. When you're in a Zoom meeting, *always* have a favorite beverage nearby. If you get frustrated, agitated, or bored, reach for it. I think of this as beverage therapy, and I have relied on beverage therapy to get me through many a meeting.

Set up your kindness. If you're switching from working in an office setting to working from home, there will be growing pains. Be kind to yourself as you transition, and as your family (or roommate or pet) gets used to this new setup. It may take a few weeks to get the hang of it. Have plans for managing frustration, disappointment, anxiety, boredom, or loneliness. Celebrate the small wins, and connect with others working from home.

28. Reclaim Your Work Friends

How we work, who we work with, and our relationships at work have all changed significantly over the years. If you're now working part-time or full-time from home, casual interactions may be limited or nonexistent. If you're back at a work site, you may find that former coworkers have moved on. Perhaps you're short-staffed or your coworkers are extra stressed. Or you may have started a new job and must learn your new responsibilities and get to know the other employees. *Breathe.*

Research shows that having friends at work is good for your mental health and well-being (Clifton and Harter 2021). Consider the following ways to develop or reclaim relationships with your coworkers and choose one to try within the next week:

Say hello and introduce yourself to the folks around you. I've noticed that the simple introduction is a vanishing art. Unless you're wearing a name tag every day, it's your responsibility to break the ice and introduce yourself to as many people in your workplace as possible. Get the other person's name and remember it for the next time you meet. An easy way to remember someone's name is to add a positive adjective before it in your mind; for example, remember Frank as *funny Frank*, Kimberly as *kind Kimberly*.

Strike up a conversation. Some of us have lost the skill of small talk, from being on our computers and phones so much and having less direct contact with others. Now is a good time to practice striking up a brief conversation with another person at work. If you feel lost or shy, that's normal. Have a few open-ended questions at the ready; for example, "What's your favorite lunch place nearby?" or "Do you have any recommendations for a local gym or workout studio?" or "What are your plans for the weekend?" or "What are your vacation plans?"

Enjoy your lunch break in the break room. I can't tell you how many years I ate my lunch in my small office, not venturing out to interact with others during my precious thirty-minute lunchbreak. I think I missed some golden opportunities to connect with my colleagues. When I finally decided to open up and interact with colleagues at the hospital where I worked, I started a monthly group meeting for us, with a focus on taking care of ourselves. I called it Consultation Lunch and Wellness—CLAW for short (pun intended). It was a relaxed way to have some time together, grab lunch, and support each other's well-being.

Compliment your work friends. It feels so good to get noticed for the work you do. In turn, let your work friends and colleagues know you see and appreciate their effort, with simple phrases like "You've done a wonderful job on that project" or "Thanks for helping me complete that assignment; it was great working with you" or "I respect your ability to get the job done on time." Small, sincere compliments go a long way to making your work relationships feel good. Don't wait to compliment someone.

Sign that card. I used to think signing an office birthday card was not that important; it felt a bit cheesy. Then I had a death in the family. Everyone in my office was so supportive, and they gave me a beautiful plant and a heartfelt card signed by everyone. It felt incredibly thoughtful, and I felt closer to the team. Since that time, I've been the one to buy the cards and make sure everyone gets a chance to write a little something. Give it a try. You might even find that you develop work friendships when you bond over celebrations and life events.

29. Give Your Desk a Little Love

Let's start with the end of the work day. It's the most important time to give your desk a little love. Your desk works hard for you. Papers everywhere, cups, snack wrappers, notepads, pens, books, folders, computer, phone, and sticky notes galore. Thank your desk for providing the environment for you to contain everything in one place and get your work done. Your desk has been there for you, like a best friend and confidante. Now it's time to give back. When you knock off work, ten minutes before you leave or close down your home office, take a look at your hardworking desk. This may sound radical, but I'd like you to clear your desk (so that you can see the surface). This means you get to:

1. Take cups (and possibly lunch containers) to the sink and rinse them out.

2. Throw away any wrappers that haven't made it into the wastebasket yet.

3. Return books to the bookshelf.

4. Store notebooks and notepads in the top drawer of your desk for easy access the next workday.

5. Collect all the sticky notes and either recycle them if they are no longer important or stick them all on one page of your notebook.

6. Put all pens and pencils in a top desk drawer. You only need one pen at a time.

7. Close all tabs on your computer that you no longer need; save important items to the desktop or designated folders.

8. Put away all papers, or shred any confidential papers that you no longer need.

9. Turn off your computer and clean your keyboard.

10. Finally, clean the surface with a great-smelling cleaner (try orange, lemon, or grapefruit) in preparation for your next work session.

Wonderful. You've just given yourself a small but mighty gift of a clear desk for the next work session. Notice what it feels like to return to your tidied-up desk. Is your mind more clear and less stressed? Your desk is ready to welcome you back. Do you feel ready to greet the next work day with renewed energy?

30. Boss Yourself Around

Think back to who your favorite boss was (or is currently). This could be a favorite boss from ten years ago or someone who is your boss now. Do you have the image in mind? What are their characteristics? What do you like best about them? Jot down a few traits that come to mind. I've listed some characteristics of my favorite bosses over the years; see if any resonate with you:

- **Energetic.** Having enough energy to tackle the most challenging of situations or assignments is such a fundamental characteristic for a good boss.

- **Supportive.** Being a beacon of support may sound simple, but many bosses lack this crucial characteristic.

- **Motivated.** You know it when you feel it. I tend to gravitate to people who are inspiring and motivated to do a good job and take pride in their work.

- **Honest.** There are some bosses that don't tell you the whole truth. When you find out they haven't been honest, work life becomes awkward, and you may understandably feel resentful.

- **Resourceful.** I've worked at more than one job that didn't provide the basic resources to the staff (like a clean environment or enough space or adequate office supplies). Does your boss provide the resources you need to get the job done?

- **Self-aware.** Such a boss is self-aware and understands how their interactions affect others. This is one of my *favorite* characteristics in bosses, and one that I treasure in my colleagues too!

- **Forward thinking.** Is your boss able to see future trends and capitalize on them? This requires the ability to think about the future and how it affects you as an employee, the business, and the bottom line.

- **Resilient.** Some bosses are great when things are going well, but it feels like it's their first day on the job when there is a work emergency or local crisis. Is yours able to handle big challenges?

- **Able to assess and reward.** Getting rewarded for a job well done just plain feels good (even if it's a small reward). It can make the difference between retaining a valuable employee—or losing them.

Add to this list any more characteristics that you love in a boss. Now take another look at the list. Which of these characteristics do you show *yourself* regularly, now that you're changing your relationship with alcohol in your life? Pick two, and be the positive boss to yourself that you need right now. Don't wait for someone else to offer you these valuable and necessary characteristics; cultivate them in yourself, and notice how you feel when you boss yourself around with admiration and kindness.

● ● ● ● ●

Take a moment to answer these questions:

What can I offer myself at work today?

What can I let go of at work today?

Reconnect with Your Work Checklist

How will you know when you've been able to truly reconnect with your work? Consider this list and see which one speaks to you. Choose one area to focus on this week:

- [ ] Practice building one boundary for wellness at work.

- [ ] Do one thing to make your home an inviting and productive place for you to work.

- [ ] Choose one activity to reclaim your work friends.

- [ ] Try one action to give your desk a little love.

- [ ] Choose one positive boss characteristic and activate it within yourself.

It's been awesome for you to give yourself time to reconnect with work. Next, we focus on savoring healthy food and drink to continue on our journey of unwinding. Yum.

Chapter 7

Savor Your Food and Drink

I'm not crazy about reality, but it's still the only place to get a decent meal.

—Groucho Marx

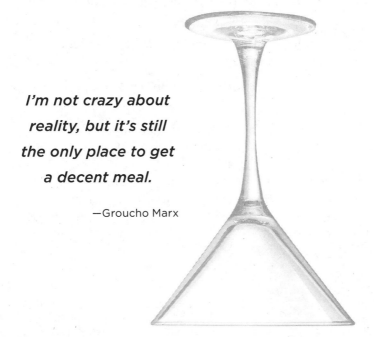

YOU MIGHT GUESS THAT DRINKING alcohol can really affect how much you eat, your food choices, and your energy to cook healthy meals for yourself. When we drink alcohol, we're more likely to eat more in general (Kwok et al. 2019), to eat less healthy foods, and to forgo taking the time to cook nutritious meals for ourself and our family.

Since alcohol is made up of ethanol—created when yeast ferments the sugars in grains (that turn into beer), fruits (that turn into wine), and vegetables (that turn into vodka and other spirits)—it tends to be dense in calories. You may recognize this cycle: You drink alcohol to deal with stress or to try to relax, and drinking impacts your sleep. Poor sleep and not feeling well may lead you to drink more, and drinking more impacts your food choices. And so it goes. But there is a way to break the cycle—by reconnecting with foods that feed your well-being, by planning what ingredients to pick up at the store, by adding vegetarian choices to your diet, and by keeping life interesting with nonalcoholic drinks or mocktails.

Let's turn our attention to taking care of your nutrition. This doesn't need to happen all at once. Take it in steps, *breathe*, and be kind to yourself along the way.

31. Reignite Your Nutrition

Don't let the word *nutrition* scare you. No white coat and clipboard here. Nutrition comes from the word *nourish*. To nourish means to give your body what it needs, when it needs it, for optimum health. Now that you're changing your relationship with alcohol, you might have different nutritional needs. When you were drinking regularly, much of your calorie intake came from alcohol. Maybe you didn't eat well, skipped eating altogether, or relied on a liquid dinner. Maybe you gravitated to salty or sugary foods. Don't let past food choices derail you from making good choices now. Once again, *breathe*.

A note on *sugar*. If you have cut down or stopped drinking alcohol recently, you may be craving sugar. Cake, donuts, cookies, ice cream, or pie suddenly seem to be calling your name. This is normal and explainable. Since giving up all the sugar that makes up most alcoholic drinks, your body and brain are looking for that next hit, adjusting to not having alcohol on board. Sugar, like alcohol, can be addictive: The more you consume, the more you want. Sugar activates dopamine in the brain, and it feels good for a short period of time, leading you to want more of that pleasurable feeling.

Try these steps when you're feeling a sugar craving. They spell SUGAR, easy to remember when you're in the middle of a craving:

S: Slow down when you feel the craving for sugar. You can always return to your awesome breathing practice.

U: Understand what you're actually feeling. Are you hungry, or thirsty (for water), angry, sad, lonely, bored, or just plain tired? It's a good idea to first be clear about how you're feeling.

G: Gain perspective. Being an observer rather than rushing in is the best way to make choices about what type of food will nourish you. What are you noticing?

A: Alternative behaviors. Sometimes doing something different or leaving the environment you're in (which may have a bunch of sweets) is the best bet. Go outside, go for a walk if you can, take a break, reach for an alternative sugar-free snack, or wait it out.

R: Reconnect to yourself with kindness. Be extra kind to yourself as you navigate the tricky terrain of understanding how sugar could be impacting you, now that you've decided not to have alcohol in your day.

Getting ahead of this sugar craving is all about preparing for it (it will happen!) and having *healthy substitutes* at the ready. Consider these options to ignite your nutrition and choose one:

● Find out what foods nourish you, what foods feel good when you eat them.

● Focus on fruits and vegetables.

● Have regular mealtimes.

● Make sure your meals are balanced.

● Drink more water.

● See if you can not eat in the three hours before bedtime and allow your brain and body to rest and recover.

● Consult a nutritionist, naturopathic doctor, or medical doctor to ask about smart, healthy food choices. (Some employer health insurance plans include visits with a dietitian.)

● Determine, with a professional's help, whether supplements would help support your health.

It's terrific that you're thinking about your nutrition and how you want to focus on a few goals. Remember to take it step by step.

32. Celebrate Small Changes

The changes you're making will be slow and steady. There is no prize for how fast you make changes to your nutrition; just keep at it. You may find you have a bit more time if you're going out less or can get up earlier without that dreaded hangover. It's good to pause and offer yourself kindness. It's also good to have a few enjoyable ways to acknowledge your mini milestones on the journey of making healthy decisions about your relationship with alcohol. You're in charge of the energy you bring to your nutritional and beverage choices. You're the CEO—Chief Energy Officer.

Don't let your small successes go unnoticed. Celebrate both small and mighty changes you're making every day to be more mindful about healthy food and drink choices. Choose one of these:

- Treat yourself to a new kitchen gadget that you'll use to cook healthy meals at home.

- Ask a friend to meet you at a local restaurant and share a dish with local flair.

- Set the table with your best dishes and silverware, light a few candles, and enjoy a home-cooked meal.

- If it is close to a holiday, be creative with your seasonal or holiday table setting to ring in the event.

- As you begin a meal, first close your eyes and say a prayer or blessing.

- Slow down at dinner and ask everyone at the table what was their win for the week.

- Pack your lunch for work or pack your family's lunch and add a kind note to make your or their day.

- Borrow new and classic cookbooks from the library. Give yourself time to look through them and get inspiration to try new recipes, then buy your own copy of your favorites.

- In your morning or evening meditation, give thanks for all you've accomplished with respect to choosing healthy food and drink.

- Make a dinner playlist of your favorite songs. Sing along as you prepare your food—extra points for knowing the lyrics! I've been inspired by Bryant Terry's beautiful *Vegetable Kingdom* (2020)—he includes music recommendations for every delicious recipe.

33. Plan Your Shopping and Prep

I used to rush to the grocery store late on Sunday afternoon, with no shopping list or plan for what I needed or was going to eat in the coming week. I'd fill my cart with the same old items that I ate every week, head to the checkout line, and hope for the best. As you can imagine, my cooking (if you can call it that) was uninspiring. Pretty much identical week to week. No exciting recipes to try, no new foods to explore. I never watched cooking shows. Yes, I had a few pretty cookbooks sitting on a shelf with sticky notes on recipes I longed to try. I never tried any of them. There was a serious disconnect between me and food.

I want you to begin to reconnect with the fun of healthy food. This requires some planning. If you're a pro at food shopping and meal planning, feel free to skip this section. But if you're anything like me and need help reconnecting with nourishing food, consider these tips and choose one to try:

- **Make sure you have good storage containers.** Glass is preferred, but use what you have as you get started. (For me, having matching colorful glass containers is a fun part of reconnecting with food.)

- **Use simple, easy-to-follow cookbooks or cooking and recipe websites—the easier the better.** Again, try the library, and ask friends for their favorites (the *Recipes* and *Food Network* websites have tons of great ideas, many with follow-along videos).

- **Take time to think about what you'd like to cook and eat in the coming week.** For some reason, this is where I fell short; I didn't realize it takes time to think about and plan meals. Ask your family what they might like too. Give yourself about an hour to go through a cookbook or watch someone cooking a recipe online. At first, choose one recipe that appeals and require minimal effort. Notice that I said *recipe*, not multiple recipes. Please start with just one new recipe at a time.

- **Make a list of needed ingredients.** Check your pantry, fridge, or freezer first; you might be surprised to find a few items waiting to be used. Make a list on your phone to consult at the grocery store. Even better, a handwritten list (on a pad, or in a small inspirational journal) slows you down a bit and makes the experience more mindful.

- **Shop for your ingredients.** If you're new to this journey, give yourself time at the grocery store; try not to rush through finding the ingredients you need. Be present and connect with the experience of taking care of yourself. Some people prefer to go to the grocery store at off-peak hours to beat the rush. Early mornings or later in the evenings might work for you. Weekdays instead of weekends also offer a bit of breathing room.

- **Plan the days you will try your new recipe.** Of course, some days are just too busy to tackle a brand-new recipe. Choose an evening when you have some extra time and you can relax in the kitchen. If you have kids old enough, you may want to include them in the prep. If your partner or roommate is interested, include them too. Or if you like to be on your own and have space in the kitchen, kick everyone out and get to it. Ask them to help with cleanup—always a crowd favorite. If you've always had a glass of wine nearby when you cooked in the past, now you will doing things a bit differently. Mix yourself a nonalcoholic drink and enjoy it as you create your new dish.

You don't have to make seven new recipes each week. Start small with just one. Savor your new creation and celebrate your success. Well done!

34. Explore the Vegetarian Approach

When I decided to reduce the meat in my diet, I wasn't ready to do it all at once. So I, like many, started by enjoying one vegetarian day each week. This choice worked for me and gave me the confidence to add another meatless day. There are lots of health benefits to including more vegetarian choices in your diet. According to the Mayo Clinic (2022), these include reducing your risk of getting heart disease, diabetes, and some types of cancers—three of the top risk factors for Americans. In addition, going vegetarian or vegan, even just in small steps, will reduce your impact on the environment. The key is to try to eat a diverse selection of plant-based foods, such as fresh fruits and vegetables, legumes, nuts, and whole grains.

It's always a good idea to touch base with a registered dietitian (some insurance plans cover this) to get help with food substitutes and meal planning. Be open to different ways of thinking about your food choices, and start with *easy* vegetarian or vegan recipes.

Here are a few options (consult with your medical professional as you make changes to your diet); choose one and see how you do:

- **One day per week eat alternatives to meat.** Set a day and assemble a list of the ingredients you need to buy in advance (and see what's already in the pantry). Have fun with it. Add a new salad for lunch and dinner; try some greens that you might not normally gravitate to, like kale, spinach, or Swiss chard. If you're including your partner and kids, make them part of the experience by asking for taste testers. Serve your new recipe on different plates.

- **Be creative with your favorite meals.** For example, if you love tacos but have always had them with chicken or beef, now is a good time to try a vegetarian version. Many of your tried-and-true recipes may be delicious with substituting hearty vegetables like squash, beans, or zucchini. Look up your favorite chef or favorite food magazine and follow along with their vegetarian recipes (take a look at the websites *Barefoot Contessa*, *Giadzy*, or *Eating Well* for great vegetarian ideas). Or borrow a vegetarian or vegan cookbook from the library.

- **Ask your vegan or vegetarian friends for help.** You might run into a wall after trying a few recipes. Recruit your friends who have been at this vegetarian game longer than you. You'd be surprised what goodies they may offer you, and they may have a few preferred sites or cool cookbooks they can steer you to for that extra inspiration.

- **Buddy up.** Even better. Link up with a like-minded friend who is starting down the vegetarian path too. Together, share recipes, meet up at local vegetarian or vegan restaurants that you've never been to (check out the *Happy Cow* online directory for vegan restaurants near you), or share a dish at a local restaurant that offers vegetarian choices. Figure out if the dish you order is something you can actually make at home.

The key here is to be inventive. As you commit to changing your relationship with alcohol, you can also commit to trying vegetarian meals. See how you feel after you've had a vegetarian meal, and keep up the great work.

35. Be Mocktail Curious

If the idea of not drinking when going out to an event, hosting family or friends at your home, or celebrating a milestone sounds daunting, perhaps it's time to become a mocktail expert. Nonalcoholic drinks are having a moment, so why not ride the wave and get good at making them for yourself? Lots of nonalcoholic choices come with cool options to make the drink special (one of my favorite sources for ingredients and kits is on the *Seedlip Drinks* website). Here are some easy ways to switch from the usual cocktails to mocktails, whether at home, when you go out, or when visiting friends:

- **Plan ahead.** What to order when going out with friends could cause a fair amount of stress. Think ahead of time about what you'd like to drink and which restaurants have beverages that appeal to you. If it's available, look at the restaurant's nonalcoholic drink menu beforehand. Make sure your restaurant choice is front and center. It's okay to prepare ahead; make it easy on yourself. After all, you're changing your habits, and it helps to be a bit more organized when you're establishing a new habit.

- **The low (or no) alcohol bar.** Quite a few bars have been popping up that serve only nonalcoholic beverages. Most zero-alcohol bars are in larger cities like Los Angeles, Chicago, New York, San Francisco, and Austin (take a look at the *Sober Bars Near Me* website to see if there might be one in your neighborhood). A second option is the sober-friendly restaurant and bar scene. These offer nonalcoholic versions of drinks you may have enjoyed when you were drinking. Give one of these a try, and ditch the morning hangover.

- **Your home bar, just better.** Having choices of nonalcoholic drinks when you're home or entertaining family and friends can be a game changer for establishing new habits. Friends and family are usually curious about what you're mixing up and will more than likely want to give your new concoctions a try. My experience is that folks like the nonalcoholic drinks I make so much they usually don't switch back to wine, beer, or cocktails. Your focus should be on connecting with others, not converting anyone. It's just nice to offer an alternative to alcohol.

- **Use the good glasses.** Don't wait to break out the nice cocktail glasses for your nonalcoholic drinks. Make each occasion special, just as you would if you were serving alcoholic beverages. And if it's just you after work, it's okay to use the fancy glasses then, too. If you don't have any special beverage glasses, save up and buy them when you have the resources (also take a look at consignment or thrift stores in your area; you'll be surprised at the gems hiding out there).

- **Try different types of nonalcoholic drinks.** The competition is fierce. There are lots of nonalcoholic drinks on the market now. The idea is catching on, so why not take advantage of it? Check out what's available in your local grocery store—they may be in the liquor section or hiding in the overflowing beverage aisle. Look online for good ideas, or ask friends what they have tried and liked. It's really about exploring new drinks and new mixers and finding out what tastes you enjoy. Having a few choices of nonalcoholic drinks will level up the playing field for you; use your imagination on this journey.

You're firmly on your way to taking better care of yourself, exploring your nutritional needs, and adding creative and delicious mocktails to your social plans and down time. I'm proud of you.

● ● ● ● ●

As you savor your food and drink, take a moment to reflect on these two questions:

What food or drink choice can I offer myself today?

What food or drink choice can I let go of today?

Savor Your Food and Drink Checklist

How will you know when you've begun to savor your food and drink in a healthy way? Look at this checklist and decide which one speaks to you. Choose one area to focus on this week:

- ☐ Make one change to reignite your nutrition for optimal well-being.

- ☐ Celebrate a small change when it comes to your food choices.

- ☐ Make one plan for your shopping and food prep.

- ☐ Choose one vegetarian meal to try this week.

- ☐ Take thirty minutes to learn about mocktails and nonalcoholic drink options and choose one mocktail to try.

Your commitment to healthy and healing food and drink alternatives is inspiring. The path you're on will lead to wonderful food and drink choices. Now we are ready to move on to your family life and begin to embrace those special people (and animals) closest to you. Here we go!

Chapter 8

Embrace Your Family

*Every time you are
tempted to react in
the same old way,
ask if you want to be
a prisoner of the past
or a pioneer of the
future.*

—Deepak Chopra

FEW THINGS IN LIFE CAUSE AS MUCH stress and tension—and joy and excitement—as our families. Whether you're close to family members or estranged from them, chances are you think about them quite a bit. Now that you have a new and improved relationship with alcohol, you may feel more tension around certain family members—and more joy around others.

If your family members are currently drinking around you when you're not drinking, notice what is happening without reacting. There may be judgment about your not drinking; jokes may be thrown your way. If you notice this happening, deflect. Do not engage in any negativity. Refocus on your healthy choices and small moments of positive connection.

Or you may experience pure joy with other family members that you may not have felt when you were drinking alcohol. Embarking on new kinds of interactions is right where you should be as you make important changes in your life.

Having new kinds of interactions can create anxiety, so I want you to take it in small steps. All the fraught family relationships don't have to be repaired right away. Things take time. *Breathe.* See if you can make this a bit easier on yourself as you heal your mind and make healthy choices going forward. As we explored in chapter 5, "Nurture Your Relationships," I'd like you to anticipate that there will be changes coming your way, both welcome changes and unwelcome ones. You have what it takes to stay connected to yourself and your values here. Let's start where you are, rebuild connections with kids, offer kindness to elders, bond with animals, and take small breaks to recharge as you embrace your family in a new way.

36. Start Where You Are

Starting exactly where you are with your family has deep roots in your well-being. It's incredibly important to give yourself a moment to be present with what is when it comes to family dynamics and family roles. Numbing out or checking out may have worked for a short time in the past, but now you're turning a corner and seeing things more clearly.

If you've decided not to drink when with your family, you're embarking on a journey that will give you a new type of freedom. Here are some ways you can start where you are as you engage with and embrace your family. Choose one of these simple PEACE thank-you strategies during any family interaction, and remember to make it easy on yourself.

- **Practice your breathing.** My all-time favorite, and it works every time. Inhale for a count of four, hold for two, and exhale for a count of four. Rest a moment at the bottom of the exhale. Try this for five good breaths. And return to it throughout your time with your family, especially if you're having a tough time. This is a great way to stay grounded.

- **Engage with what's healthy in your family members.** Notice how well someone is doing, and say so. Focus on the good you see in someone's mental, physical, or spiritual health. You can say something like "I'm impressed with how far you've come in solving that problem." Comment on how important your relationship is to that family member; perhaps "I'm so happy to have you in my life." Put your phone away, make eye contact, stay in the moment, and smile.

- **Accept people where they are.** Being in the moment and accepting exactly where someone happens to be is an ongoing practice. There is no need to fix, change, convince, or force anything or anyone right now. No solutions are needed. Not needing to find an instant solution frees you up to focus on the here and now.

- **Create a compassionate space.** If you're going through a rough patch, or your family member is, be kinder and more compassionate than usual. Find space to connect if you think that would provide you both with deeper healing. Sometimes just being quiet in the same room with your family member is all that is needed. Practice moments of quiet with another person nearby. This practice includes kids, too!

- **Exit with love.** There is nothing wrong with excusing yourself and leaving a gathering early. Leaving early allows you to redirect your energy for other connections, relationships, or upcoming projects. Let your family members know that you will be leaving a bit early, and tell them you appreciate them. Be clear in your communication, and try not to apologize for taking care of yourself. If you'd like to set up another time to get together, you can do it before you exit.

- **Thank-you notes.** Little notes of connection go a long way in keeping family relationships in a place of gratitude. Texting is nice, but an actual card might be a bit nicer. Let the person know you're thinking about them and that you value the relationship. In your thank-you note, you might write "Thank you for taking time for us to connect. I cherish our relationship and will continue to make space for it to flourish. You're one of the most important people in my life." What does it feel like to write these words or other words of connection? What would it feel like to receive a note like this one?

As you continue your daily mindfulness practice, include those family interactions in the mix. Reflect on how you're feeling and changing, now that your mind is a bit less cloudy.

37. Rebuild Connections with Kids

If you have children in your life and have been feeling a bit disconnected from them over the past few months, this is a good time to see if there are some new ways to renew your connection. Whoever they are (your own children, nieces or nephews, neighborhood kids, or your friends' kids), let's see if you can refocus on them and offer them the best parts of yourself now. When you were drinking or drinking to excess, you may have unknowingly lost touch with the little moments of reunion. Alcohol has a tricky way of blocking these little moments. You may have felt bored, frustrated, or overwhelmed; you might not have felt anything at all. You may have used alcohol to cope with the stresses of being a parent or caretaker. That is the past; let's not focus on that now. Now is all about being the person, parent, or caretaker you want to be, offering your healthy self to your family, and finding innovative ways to manage the stress that is a natural part of growth.

Part of the experience of giving up alcohol is realigning with yourself and choosing healthy behaviors for yourself. Or perhaps revisiting old behaviors that used to be second nature when you were feeling great. It's about being present. Here are a few ways to reconnect with kids, whether they are little kids, young adults, or full-on adults. Reflect on how you feel with the kids in your life, and choose one of these to try:

- **Play often.** I hope I'm not stating the obvious, but many of us have lost touch with the idea of just playing without any agenda. Spend thirty minutes with the phone turned off, free to play, just goof around, tell jokes, and enjoy whatever spontaneous fun appeals to you.

● **Explore new places together.** Researching places that you haven't been to yet, then exploring them together, is another exciting way to connect. Plan to visit the new place you've found, take photos if you'd like, and have a "best photo" contest. You'll get to know what the kid likes (beyond their routine of smartphone, TV, or video games).

● **Ask questions and listen.** Along with asking good questions about how they are doing and what is new, ask what they do to have a good time. You can also ask about how they have handled a recent challenging experience. Their answers might surprise you. Remember, you don't have to fix anything or solve any problem; just listen and enjoy the moments of togetherness.

● **Be quiet together.** This may seem odd, but being in the same space with someone in quality quiet time has a profound effect on connection. Although each of you will be doing different things—say, homework and office work—there is still an important connection happening and a deep feeling of safety.

● **Cook or bake together.** Many of us have been cooking and eating at home a lot more. Up to twenty-one meals a week can feel overwhelming for just about anyone.

Take the opportunity to look up recipes together. You might be surprised what each of you like—and your tastes may have changed over the course of the months spent eating lots of meals at home. Get your aprons on and get cooking or baking.

Now that you've initiated reconnection with the kids in your life, it's time to focus on the elders in your life or in your community.

38. Offer Kindness to Elders

There are certain cultures where elders are truly respected and admired. (Unfortunately, the U.S. doesn't seem to be one of them.) In Japan, for example, the sixtieth year of life is called *kanreki*, and it's a celebration of rebirth. According to Japanese culture, this is a time to prioritize goals and clarify directions. It's nice to know that there is a positive, life-affirming way to think about our elders.

Here are a few ways you can offer kindness to elders, which in turn will give you a case of the feels. Choose one and see how you do:

- **Call your parents or grandparents.** If this is something you already do, bravo. For those who may have slacked off on calling your parents, grandparents, or another elder that you may have lost touch with, why not do it this week? If you've only called with a drink in your hand, now you'll get to experience the connection sober. Grab a cup of tea, sit back in a comfy chair, relax. You will brighten someone's day and feel close again.

- **Volunteer at a senior activity center or senior home.** There are usually a few senior centers or homes in every town, big or small. Look into the volunteer opportunities available at your local senior center. Even just a few hours a week can have a positive impact on their health and on your mood.

- **Help an elder neighbor with their lawn or plant care.** Sometimes gardens get short shrift when people are overwhelmed with taking care of themselves and the inside of their homes. And in colder regions, each winter can bring lots of snow that needs to be shoveled. Can you offer to help care for the outside of a neighbor's home?

- **Volunteer for Meals on Wheels.** This organization provides older adults, their families, and other at-risk people with home-delivered meals and helps with social isolation. In 2019, 223 million meals were provided to 2.4 million older adults. Nine million seniors in America face the threat of hunger—that's a lot of at-risk people who need this resource. The organization is always looking for volunteers to help deliver food, typically during the lunch hour; there are other volunteer opportunities that may work with your work schedule. Take a look at their website and see if this experience is a match for you.

- **Offer to drive an elder to the doctor or other appointment.** If you have a car and the resources to buy gas, is driving an elderly person to their appointment something you'd like to do? It may require waiting a bit, so set aside a few hours a week for this. Bring a favorite book with you if you'll have to wait. And offer emotional support on the drive to and from the appointment.

- **Take an elder to an exercise, yoga, or meditation class.** Staying mentally and physically vibrant is all about movement and mindfulness. See if there are

classes offered in your community that may be a perfect
fit for older folks.

If there are other acts of kindness that you can think of that
would connect you to your elders, don't be shy. Your good ideas and
reaching out will make all the difference in how you feel in sobriety.
Great job! I'm impressed with your generous spirit.

39. Bond with Animals

According to recent research (Insurance Information Institute 2022), 70 percent of all households in the United States own a pet: 45.3 million have a cat and a whopping 69 million have a dog. But we don't need statistics to acknowledge that our pets are family. During the stress of the pandemic's first year, from March 2020 to May 2021, one in five people acquired a cat or a dog. Animals are important companions; they have special ways to calm us down, improve our mood, and help us exercise by walking or playing with them.

The Veteran's Administration conducted research taking veterans with serious mental health conditions out to visit with animals in a variety of local animal environments in the community to see if their mental health conditions would improve. Not only did their conditions get noticeably better, but they were also better able to interact with other people on the outings. The veterans also reported feeling better when they interacted with each other and the animals. Hence, animals became recognized as icebreakers for social interactions (Pollock, Williams, and Gomez 2017). It's nice to know the power animals have to help strengthen our well-being. See if animals can be icebreakers for you and your interactions with others.

Choose one of these ways to include animals as part of your healing journey:

- **Spend time with your pet.** No need to complicate things here. Just hang with your furry family member. Watch a movie together, read a book, work in your home office space, play, take a walk, be mindful of your connection, and appreciate the time together.

- **Get out to the zoo or aquarium.** Find your local zoo or aquarium and plan a family visit. Take the tours and learn about the animals. You will feel like a little kid again, and this is a good thing.

- **Find an animal sanctuary.** I'm happy to say that I visited Alligator Alley in Georgia, a place where the animals roam free and the people stay in their cars. It was amazing, and I gained a new respect for those beautiful alligators. See if there is a special place for wild animals in your area, and go check it out.

- **Volunteer at a shelter.** If you wish to connect with animals who need extra help, this may be an appealing activity. If you cannot work in a shelter, perhaps you can donate money or items for animals in need. On a smaller scale, you can donate your gently used clean towels to your local animal hospital. Every little bit helps.

- **Take photos of animals in nature.** Slow down and spot animals outside. I'm lucky enough to see eagles, hawks, cranes, herons, ducks, and geese outside my back patio. My photos aren't always the greatest, but the mindful slowing down to observe these awe-inspiring birds is a beautiful way to connect with wild animals from a distance.

- **Plan a bigger animal adventure.** If you have the resources and love animals, there are lots of trips available for animal lovers. It's a fun trip to plan with your family or those closest to you.

I'm so happy you're including animals on your healing journey. Time with animals is never wasted, and there are usually some cool surprises in store for you.

40. Take Small Breaks to Recharge

Recharging in the middle of family life is just what the doctor ordered. It can be exhausting to be with family members while you're making the shift to not drinking alcohol. That is why taking small breaks is so important for you now. And these breaks don't have to be intricate or expensive. I'm not talking about a vacation in the Bahamas; I'm talking about *moments of recharge* that you can definitely do almost anywhere and with anyone you happen to be with.

Here are a few ways to give yourself small breaks when you're in the company of your family. They spell out SMALL, because even small breaks go a long way to recharging your batteries. Choose one of these for this week:

- **Sneak outside.** Get a breath of fresh air for a few minutes. This has a great way of grounding you so you can get back to your family reinvigorated. While you're outside, look around, notice your surroundings, feel the sun and wind, say a little prayer of gratitude, and breathe.

- **Make a cup of tea.** Many teas that we might take for granted have amazing healing properties, including reducing stress. Teas for destressing include mint, chamomile, lavender, rose, and matcha. Add a bit of honey or lemon if you'd like. Make sure you have a nice selection of teas on hand when visiting family or when family visits you.

- **Activate your affirmations.** Affirmations are simple phrases you can repeat over and over as a way to rewire your brain—phrases like "I am calm when interacting with others" or "Focusing on my healing helps my relationships." Or create a few affirmations of your own. If you've been beating yourself up about drinking, now is a good time to add consistent, positive, healing affirmations to your day.

- **Listen to music.** Don't underestimate the benefit of melting into calming background music when you're with your family. I'm a big fan of the vocal artistry of Roberta Flack, Norah Jones, Sade, Carole King, Jackson Browne, Diana Krall, and Michael Bublé. These or other favorite artists will infuse bright energy and relaxation into your space.

- **List your goals.** Remind yourself of your goals with your family to recenter yourself. Simple goals, like *I'm going to connect with my mother about her new friend* or *I'm going to laugh with my brother about something from the past* or *I'm going to share a recipe with my aunt* are all you need. Keep your family connection goals easy and achievable.

Please don't complicate things here. Simple and calm is always better as you navigate ways of being with your family (and they navigate ways of being with you) without drinking alcohol. It will get easier, the more experience you have under your belt, and you will continue to find genuine ways to embrace your family.

● ● ● ● ●

Answer these questions with honesty and respect for creating deeper connections with family:

What can I offer my family member today?

What can I let go of in my family today?

Embrace Your Family Checklist

How will you know when you've done what is needed to reunite and reconnect with your family? Take a look at this checklist and choose one activity to complete this week:

- ☐ Think of one way to embrace the idea of starting where you are.

- ☐ Choose one way to reconnect with kids.

- ☐ Pick one way to offer kindness to elders.

- ☐ Create one experience where you bond with animals.

- ☐ Commit to one way you can take a small break to recharge.

I hope you're feeling the benefits of your journey through these simple tips from the heart. Let's turn our attention now to another important area of being well without turning to alcohol: respect for your money. This one requires an extra dose of kindness!

Chapter 9

Respect Your Money

Wealth flows from energy and ideas.

—William Feather

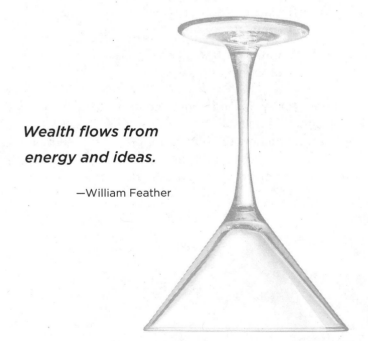

I DON'T WANT YOU TO HAVE A TUG-OF-WAR with yourself about money. With you on one side and money on the other, pushing and pulling through life. Here we'll be going a bit deeper to help you understand your relationship with money.

If the idea of respecting your money is a foreign concept, you're not alone. Many of us blow through cash without any idea of where it all goes. Or, if we do know where it goes, we are shocked that we don't seem to have enough for the things we need. The pressure to buy, buy, buy is intense. The pressure to keep up with your friends, family, work colleagues, and social media is constant. Now that you're making other important changes in your life regarding alcohol use, you get to have a more mindful approach to your relationship with money. Together, we are going to set the stage to review your finances with love, find ways to decrease your spending a bit each day, uncover ideas to pay off your debt, learn new ways to earn money that you might not have thought of, and plan for some well-deserved fun along the way. The key is to have a financial goal that you feel good about working toward, whether it is paying down your debt, saving for a special purchase, having more savings in your account, or planning for your retirement. Go easy on yourself here, and *breathe*.

41. Review Your Finances with Love

Few things cause people more dread than actually taking an honest look at their finances and spending habits. Whether you're struggling paycheck to paycheck or have a bit of money in savings, this is a great opportunity to pull back the covers and see what is really going on with your money. We will be taking a look at what you're spending each month. And we are going to get real about how much you've been spending on alcohol. *Breathe*. Having this information will be empowering.

It's important to give yourself love all along the way. There is no judgment here. Like me, you may never have learned how to manage your money. When I was growing up, my parents never talked about money with us. It was a taboo subject in the house, but it felt like there was a lot of tension about not having enough. If your family was a bit like mine, you can change things for the better. If your finances are tied in with a partner or spouse, please invite them to join you. Here are a few mindful tips on reviewing your finances and taking care of yourself along the way. Let's get started.

1. **Set time aside to focus on your finances.** It may not all happen in one sitting. Give yourself at least one hour a week to focus on where you are right now financially. This is the time you will begin to review your financial choices.

2. **Make a cup of tea or coffee.** It sounds simple, but this act of treating yourself to a hot beverage establishes an

environment of calmness and safety as you begin this process. The caring messages you give yourself now set the stage for how your relationship with money changes for the better.

3. **Close your eyes and take three deep, cleansing breaths.** Breathing helps you connect with the present moment. Being in the present is the first step to self-awareness about money.

4. **When you're ready, look at your bank or credit card statement.** Offer your bank or credit card statements some love and kindness. Thank them for being there for you, for taking care of your money business.

5. **Write in your journal what you're spending money on.** Now the fun part. Make columns for each important expense category. Expenses are your necessities—your *needs*. These are the areas you will be tracking (with love) on a monthly basis (adapted from http://www.nerdwallet .com):

    -   **Housing.** This includes rent or mortgage payment, renter's or homeowners' insurance, property taxes, home repairs and improvements, landscaping, and other home needs.

    -   **Health care.** This includes health insurance premiums, copays and deductibles, medications, and supplements.

    -   **Food expenses.** This includes groceries and toiletries.

- **Transportation.** This includes public transportation; car payments, insurance, repairs, and gas.

- **Child care.** This includes monthly childcare, babysitting, kids' classes, and summer camps.

- **Pet expenses.** This includes food, vet visits, medications, toys, and pet sitting.

- **Utilities.** This includes electricity and gas, water, garbage pickup, internet, cable, cell phone, and landline.

- **Loans and other payments.** This includes student loans, child support, alimony, and personal loans.

Next, track your *wants*. These are the items that you like but perhaps are not necessary right now. These may be extra expenses and a great place to reassess and scale back a bit.

- **Clothing, shoes, and jewelry.** Be honest here; these costs add up quickly.

- **Eating and drinking out.** Include your coffee habit here, and create a separate column for alcohol expenditures. No judgment, just data.

- **Events.** Movies, concerts, and sporting events (include any gambling here).

- **Fitness.** Gym memberships, online or in-person fitness classes.

- **Travel.** Transportation to the airport, airline or rail tickets, hotels or Airbnbs, booked tours, and rental cars.

- **Cable or streaming services.** Add up all these expenses here, including video games.

- **Self-care:** Massages or other bodywork, facials, haircuts, manicures and pedicures.

- **Home needs:** Plants, furniture and lighting, kitchen items, bedding, home office supplies.

- **Books, music, magazine, and podcast subscriptions.** Include your book buying and all subscriptions.

It's important to get the big picture and see where you're spending your hard-earned money. Next, let's take a look how you can begin to change your spending habits with a lot of love.

42. Decrease Spending Today

The best way to begin to decrease spending is to first look at the *want* list you compiled and choose one area to focus on. For example, look at your cable or streaming services. I'm probably not the first person to feel overwhelmed with the number of cable TV channels I somehow accumulated over the years. In my house, sports, movies, and home improvement shows rule. It feels like new channels are regularly offered (these channels always have a plus + after their name, making us feel like we are missing out if we don't buy the plus +).

Now, instead of Sports + or Home +, or Movie +, we are going to focus on Don't Spend + or Savings +. We have to talk about wants and needs here. Decide what you can let go of, and be honest with yourself. If you share the TV with your family, they get a vote too. When you take something away or give something up, it's usually a good idea to replace it with a healthy alternative. Here are some tried and true (and easy) ways to decrease your spending; choose one that works best for you:

- **Can it wait a day (CIWAD)?** Before you spend money on anything, ask yourself this all-important question. Then revisit the item the next day, and see if you still need it. The savings on this question alone are limitless.

- **Bring your lunch to work** and see if you can eat outdoors or eat with a work colleague to make it less humdrum. Make lunch for your whole family and reap extra savings of about $2,500 a year.

- **Ditch bottled water** and purchase an inspiring reusable stainless steel or glass bottle and invest in a water filter. Savings here could be about $250 a year. The environment will send you a thank-you card for this one.

- **Forgo buying gifts for a year** and find creative ways to celebrate birthdays, anniversaries, weddings, and holidays. Thoughtful cards, plant clippings, homemade goodies, or books you've read and can pass on are great ideas. The list is endless. Savings depends on your current gifting habits, but could be hundreds of dollars a year.

- **Make your own coffee.** A cup of coffee out in the world is around $5.00, and if you, like most of us, have a serious coffee habit, that's over $100 per month or $1,200 per year. Invest in a good coffee maker and pocket the rest of the cash.

- **Visit your local library.** I love books and have spent quite a lot of money on them over many years. As an author I felt like I was supporting my tribe. My husband recommended we get library cards. You can go onto your library's website, find the books you want, and put them on hold, renew the books you love, and return the books that don't quite cut it. If you used to buy a few books each month, you will be saving about $500 a year. Check out your local used book store to reap some extra savings.

- **Slash your subscriptions.** Taking a long hard look at the subscriptions you pay for every month may be a wake-up call. I was getting magazines each month that I had no time (or desire) to read. See if you can cancel anything that no longer brings you enjoyment, and find similar topics in online magazines or blogs for free. You might be able to save more than $300 a year.

- **Reduce your water use.** I remember reading about a celebrity who timed her showers and got them down to five minutes max. If everyone in the house lowers their time in the shower by a few minutes, this could help decrease both the water and the heating bills. We installed an energy-efficient water heater in our current home and saved over $400 per year. Look for rebates and tax credits for any energy-efficient appliances.

- **Not drinking today.** Money you used to spend on alcohol either by going out or drinking at home adds up fast. Some people can pocket upward of $2,000 a year.

Once you've put in place one or more of these easy habits, you can move that money you save into paying off your debt and adding to your savings account. Just on these nine ways to save, you can potentially save over $7,500 a year. Great job!

43. Pay Off Debt and Save

Credit cards, student loans, car payments, mortgage payments, and personal loans. There is no shortage of debt that we all carry. The burden can sometimes feel quite heavy, and the stress may have caused you to turn to alcohol to just not think about it. Now that you're clear-headed without the strain of hangovers, it's a great time to take a closer look at your debt. Being honest with your debt is the first step in creating a plan to tackle it. *Breathe*. When you're ready to get serious about paying off your debt, here is what financial experts recommend. Remember to be extra kind to yourself as you move through this process. Choose one of these and reflect on how you're doing:

- **Make a list of everything you owe.** Seeing everything on paper is the first step to getting clear about the direction you want to take.

- **Review your budget.** What money is coming in and what is going out is important information to have.

- **See if you can lower your bills.** Many experts advise calling up your loan company and asking them to lower your interest rates. Don't be afraid to try this step; you might be pleasantly surprised.

- **Don't be late.** This may be obvious, but one of the best ways to pay down debt is to not get charged late fees or overdraft fees. Pay every bill on time (or early, if possible).

- **Revisit your side hustle.** With a clear goal in mind to pay down your debt, getting a side job on a temporary basis may get you to your goal faster. My side hustle was teaching yoga on the weekends. It helped pay off my student loan.

- **Ask for help.** Going to a credit counselor may be the right decision for you if you feel overwhelmed and are not sure you can get a handle on your finances. (Some employers offer credit counseling as part of your benefits package.)

- **Pay off your smallest debt first.** Pay the minimum on all of your other debts. Then pay the extra you have from paying off your smallest debt toward the next highest debt.

When I was working as a vocational psychologist for the VA Hospital, I worked with many veterans who didn't have a savings account. It was a surprise to me. They just didn't think they had enough money to put into a savings account. I'm here to tell you, you *do* have enough to start a savings account. And if you haven't put money in your savings account for a long time, now is the time to start back up. Putting a little in your savings account each month will definitely add up. And the money you're not spending on alcohol and going out for cocktails can easily make it over to your savings. See if you can start with $20 a week. In a year, that adds up to over $1,000 in savings.

If finances are a weak area for you, it's a good idea to take a class on finance. There are usually free or low-cost classes offered at your local community center, at your local college, or online. You are worth it, and you will experience the benefits for many years to come.

44. Learn to Earn

Sometimes one of the best ways to tackle money issues is to see if you can earn more money at the same job or find other ways to earn a bit of extra income. The thought of asking for a raise at work makes most of us nervous. How do you go about asking for a raise without stressing yourself out? Have a plan, and write down the main points you want to address with your boss. Generally speaking, employers do want to take care of their good employees. The average pay raise is 3 percent of your current salary; 4 to 5 percent is a great raise. *Breathe.* Here are a few pointers to think about and move forward on (adapted from Martin 2022). The pointers spell out RAISE, so you can remember them when you're in a meeting with your employer:

R: Review your accomplishments. No time to be humble here; write down your accomplishments over the past year. Outline how your work has gone above and beyond to significantly impact the business. Use specific numbers and percentages to make your point. Be as detailed as possible.

A: Assess the competition. Researching what typical salaries are in your field is critical to developing a good plan to ask for a raise. Some helpful sites to get started on your research are the *Salary* and *Payscale* websites. Make sure your résumé is 100 percent up to date and includes your most recent work. I had a habit of updating my résumé monthly (and dating it at the bottom of the last page) to keep track of my current work and accomplishments.

I: In it for them. We all want to know what's in it for us; it's just part of being human. This is where you outline how you can *improve* the company going forward. Unpack your goals for the company, how you plan to achieve these goals, and how they benefit the company as a whole.

S: Sure of yourself. Being sure-footed when you set up an appointment and go in to talk to your boss is definitely in your best interests. You've worked hard, and you deserve to be proud of yourself and what you've given to the company. You've prepared for this, and you have the facts to back up your request. Use your breathing skills to keep yourself calm.

E: Efforts in writing. Write a one-page summary of your raise request, the comparable pay ranges for the work you do, and the benefits your company will get from your continued high level of commitment. Bring your updated résumé in case your boss needs a reminder of your professional accomplishments. Give your boss a copy of your accomplishment summary too.

Be sure to check back with your boss within a reasonable time frame; two weeks is usually a reasonable period for your request to be reviewed. Of course, it is not unusual to get a no on the first try. Don't be disheartened. Find out what you can do at work to be considered for a raise in the near future. Be grateful and calm. If and when you get a yes, congratulations! Choose healthy nonalcohol ways to celebrate this milestone.

Along with asking for a raise, the other way to earn more cash is to find extra work. Take it from someone who has always had more than one job her entire life! I like the idea of having multiple sources of income. Take a look at a few ways you can supplement your income and choose one:

- Write blogs or articles for pay.

- Teach a class.

- Sell your clothes or household goods you no longer want.

- Work a less-demanding job on the weekends.

- Tutor a student.

- Get paid to answer surveys.

- Join a delivery service.

- Sign up to be a voting poll worker.

- Pick up seasonal work.

Think of other less taxing ways to make a bit of extra cash so that you can pay down your debt. Well done! You're on your way to creatively tackling your debt and remaining compassionate with yourself along the way.

45. Plan Low-Cost or No-Cost Fun

Now that we have reviewed your finances with love and respect, found small ways to decrease your spending, focused on paying down your debt and saving some money, and found other ways to earn money, let's plan for some low-cost or no-cost fun. Since you've decided to reevaluate your relationship with alcohol, there may be new ways to bring enjoyment into your life that won't break the bank. Figure out how much money you were spending on alcohol each month and begin to reallocate some of that to fun. Choose one of these and go for it:

- **Get a library card and explore books again.** This tip from #42 bears repeating. You might be surprised what your local library has in store for you. Books, music, games, and magazines that you'd normally buy are now available for borrowing. The library also offers computer classes, book clubs, and a great sense of community.

- **Look online for room inspirations, then pick a room to rearrange your furniture.** Moving furniture is a great way to move stagnant energy around in your home, and it will definitely change your mood for the better.

- **Ask a friend to go on a walk, and choose a fresh location.** This also dips into the relationship zone and the exercise zone. Three for one!

- **Learn about investing in stocks.** Some employers offer information on this. Investigate online or ask a close friend for a reputable company.

- **Take a class at your local community center.** Many areas have learning centers; dip a toe in and see how it goes. Choose classes with a mind open to exploring topics and activities that you've never tried before.

- **Organize a potluck.** Food is a universally popular way to bring the low-cost fun. Stir up your favorite recipes and invite folks over.

- **Volunteer to tutor a child or teenager.** Some kids may have fallen behind in school or struggle with a particular subject; their parents may welcome your offer to help.

- **Walk or ride a bike around your neighborhood.** Check out interesting streets to gain a fresh outlook on your home base.

There are so many low-cost or no-cost entertaining things to do. See if you can add a few ideas to this list. This is where you can be creative and explore new ways to be in your community.

I'm impressed that you've decided to focus on your financial well-being and have some fun along the way. You are worth it; don't give up. I know you will experience great benefit when you love and respect your money goals. You will have less stress and be able to focus on what is truly important in your life.

● ● ● ● ●

Take a few moments to answer these questions with honesty and kindness toward
yourself and your money:

*What respectful money choice can I
offer myself today?*

*What money choice can I let go of
today?*

Respect Your Money Checklist

How will you know when you have begun to respect and appreciate your money? Consider this checklist and choose one area to focus on this week:

- ☐ Review one area of your finances, with love, for optimal well-being.
- ☐ Choose one area to decrease your spending today.
- ☐ Plan one way to pay off debt.
- ☐ Give yourself one way to learn to earn.
- ☐ Plan one low-cost or no-cost fun activity.

Wonderful! We are up to the final chapter, which brings your attention to celebrating your beautiful spirit. Check in with yourself and see how you're feeling as you stick the landing of the great decisions you're making and move more fully into your healthy self.

Chapter 10

Celebrate Your Spirit

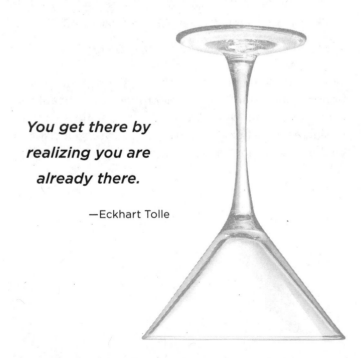

You get there by realizing you are already there.

—Eckhart Tolle

WHEN YOU GIVE UP SOMETHING THAT may have been a part of you and is certainly a part of our culture, like drinking alcohol, it is guaranteed that you will feel *a loss*. The grief is not just for the alcohol itself, but for all the things alcohol may have given you, like a social life, comfort, celebration, and the chance to unwind and fall asleep. You were attached to alcohol, perhaps for many years. Now you're in the strange and perhaps uncomfortable place of not drinking. It's like being on a new planet, with new feelings, new ways of interacting with others, and lots of activities you may never have tried before. Give yourself some room to celebrate your spirit.

Once you've figured out ways to take care of yourself, challenges will arise. Like being at a holiday party sober, celebrating without alcohol, or interacting with your friends without a glass of wine or beer in your hand. Part of this journey is to build your confidence to navigate the world without feeling shame or embarrassment. What do you want to create space for in your life? This is where reconnecting with your spirit comes in. When I talk about spirit, I am really talking about your core values and integrity, who you are deep down, what energy you're putting out into the world, and how you find quiet and joy in the everyday of life.

Let's focus on rebalancing in the here and now, getting back into art, engaging in mutual support, giving back a little at a time, and finding joy in everyday moments.

46. Rebalance in the Here and Now

Ordinary, everyday experiences and all the feelings that go with them are part of your inner work. You've been able to feel resilient in lots of different settings. Even the difficult emotions, like anger, sadness, fear, or boredom, have turned out to be your friends as you make your way down this path. Noticing even your difficult feelings can link you back to the present. You have two feet on the ground, rebalancing what is happening in the here and now. Whatever is happening to you is actually happening *for* you. And as you reassess your relationship with alcohol, you will also be realigning with parts of you that may have been dormant or shut down for some time. It's time for a wake-up call.

The opposite of rebalancing yourself in the here and now is being resistant to the here and now. Fighting what you don't like takes a lot of energy that you might be able to put into something for your higher good. Here are some simple ways to give up the fight and reconnect with the here and now:

- **Breathe.** Let your inhale and your exhale be smooth and unrestricted. Return to your breath when the outside world seems overwhelming or confusing. Breathe down into any areas of the body that feel unusually tight and stiff (like your lower back).

- **Observe.** Take a look at what is right in front of you, without judgment and without trying to change it. If someone is annoying you, notice it without trying to fix it or teach the person a lesson. Get grounded by looking around the space you are in, and be curious about how you are in the space.

- **Feel.** One of the hardest things to do when you remove alcohol from the equation is to feel what you're actually feeling without blocking, sidestepping, or overthinking it. Your feelings are real and legitimate, and they are temporary.

- **Honor.** Respect and honor where you are right now, in this moment. Try not to dwell on the past or predict the future. Sometimes when you focus on the past, depression has a way of descending on you. And when you think about the future, anxiety sometimes floats to the surface.

Where you are right now is exactly where you should be. Explore the energy you're bringing to the present moment. Notice how you're able to calm down, not judge yourself or others, and use your breath to center yourself. I see good things happening for you as you practice these skills every day.

47. Get Your Art On

Art, in all its forms, offers the deepest connection you can make to your spirit. Creating art—making music, writing, dancing, taking photographs, sculpting, knitting, painting, singing, performing, making jewelry, cooking, building, doing carpentry, and more—all are designed to express your inner spirit. You may find that once you remove alcohol from your life, your inner artistic world opens up in fascinating ways. Many recovery centers across the country include art therapy as a way to reconnect with healing and to engage mindfully in the creative process. Sometimes words don't convey what you want to communicate, or it's just difficult to find the right words for what you're experiencing. Art bridges the gap and allows you to communicate and be fully yourself.

The tricky part is to not judge yourself or your art. Think of your creations as just expressions of your life experience unfolding. These creations are not designed to be sold or even looked at by anyone else. Art is a way for you to heal and feel mentally and emotionally well.

Here are a few simple ways to reengage with your creative side and soothe stress. Choose one and begin your creative journey:

- **Take an art or writing class.** Look in your local community for low-cost or free art or writing classes. If you cannot find an in-person class, see if there is an online class that appeals to you.

- **Look for low-cost art supplies.** Finding low-cost art supplies takes some patience. Wait for monthly or holiday sales at your local art store. Start small and build your supplies up slowly.

- **Create a space to create.** Having your own space dedicated just to art is a luxury indeed. See if you can designate a corner of a room, a space in the garage, or another small space just for creating.

- **Go out to look at art.** Art can be found in so many places, not just museums. Look outside for art on the side of buildings, in flower arrangements, and in store window decorations. Go to a book reading at a local bookstore. Be curious and open-minded.

- **Watch documentaries of artists.** Some of the best ideas I get for exploring my creativity come from watching other artists and writers talk and commit to their craft. Take a look at the top artist documentaries and dive in.

- **Read about art.** Reading about art and artists is a fun way to connect with the creative journey. Those coffee-table books you might have acquired just for show in the past can now be opened up and explored. Reading memoirs or biographies of artists and writers is a wonderful way to get inside the craft.

- **Listen to podcasts by or about artists.** Many podcasts now uncover artists' life paths. If you feel stuck, pick your favorite artist or writer and search by name for an interview that you can listen to.

- **Give yourself time to create.** Setting aside time to reengage with your creativity is a necessity. Don't beat yourself up for procrastinating. Think of it as a pause, then get right back to your art and create.

- **Make art a daily practice.** Anything that you make into a daily habit will become second nature to you. Carve out time each day to engage in the habit of creating; you will not be disappointed.

- **Buddy up to work on an art project.** My favorite time writing my previous books, *The Mindfulness Workbook for Addiction* and *The Gift of Recovery*, was my frequent connections with my coauthor, marriage and family therapist Julie Kraft. If you have someone you'd like to buddy up with to do an art or writing project, ask away and see where the project takes you.

Now that you've recommitted to art as an expression of healing your mind without alcohol, keep it up. Dedicate time to your craft and see how you feel moving forward.

48. Engage in Mutual Support

Support is a two-way street. There are times when you'll need support and times when you'll give support to others, especially as you find your footing in an alcohol-free lifestyle. Look around or ask around for like-minded people. Find one or two who share your interests and reach out to offer your support.

If, for example, you're writing an article for a magazine, are there others you can reach out to in a local writing circle? Is there a mothers' group that doesn't drink alcohol that you can connect with? Is there a local class you'd like to invite someone to? Or is there someone who likes to explore new areas of town that you can invite along? Look online for alcohol-free events in your area. Ask around at work to see if anyone is interested in getting a bite to eat, and have a few nearby spots that you can try. I know this will feel awkward at first, but venture out. This is about getting out of your comfort zone and leading with your heart.

Offering support to a friend, colleague, or acquaintance may be second nature to you. But in case you're out of practice, here are a few ways to jump back into quality connections. Choose one of these with an old or new friend in the next week:

- **Provide a space and time to talk.** Having a safe and inviting environment to connect for uninterrupted minutes is heaven on earth. Even if you're connecting online, see if you can carve out a quiet place and thirty minutes.

- **Listen without thinking about what you want to say next.** Listening is an art form; it takes practice and patience. The more you listen, the better you become at it. Remember to *breathe*. The key here is to have no agenda and no quick fixes.

- **Ask open-ended questions.** It's best to start your questions with phrases like "How did you handle that?" or "What was that like for you?" Try not to ask "why" questions; these can sometimes feel judgmental.

- **Offer support and encouragement.** A few simple yet powerful words of encouragement to someone who's having a hard time go a long way. Expressions like "I have faith in you" or "I've seen you handle this before" or "I know you will figure this out" can work wonders in supporting your friend without trying to impose your own solutions.

- **Suggest a resource.** If a book, podcast, TV show, or online resource comes to mind, this is a great way to show that you understand what your friend or colleague is experiencing. Send them the resource link with a little note that says "thinking of you."

- **Laugh together.** Finding humor in challenges is an easy way to take the edge off. Connect with laughter—perhaps by watching a comedy together to lighten things up.

- **Reflect on the experience.** Ending a chat with a positive comment about how it felt for you to connect is the best way to bond with another person. "I'm really happy we connected today; I appreciate our friendship" is really all you'll need to get started.

When you need support, see if that same person is available, and ask them to set time aside to talk. Asking for the support you need when you need it may feel uncomfortable at first, but it is part of your growth. And doing it without alcohol in the mix is incredibly powerful. People love to feel needed, so don't hesitate to ask for help.

49. Give Back—A Little Goes a Long Way

Now that you're feeling better and better each day, you have a fresh opportunity to give back in small ways. What does your neighborhood or community need right now? How can you tap into the energy of where you live? For instance, in my community my husband and I once waited two hours in line to vote in the primary elections. Lots of people in line ahead of us could not wait that long and had to go back to work. We saw with our own eyes a lot of missed votes. When we finally got to the front of the line, we saw that there were only three poll workers checking people in. We made the decision then and there that we could help a little by signing up to be poll workers to help decrease some of the burden of too many voters and too few poll workers. That's not going to fix the problem, but it's a small way to give back to our new community.

There are lots of creative ways to give your energy to a cause or issue you believe in or that is important to you. If you want to volunteer but don't know exactly where the greatest need is, take a look at the *Volunteer Match* website (some you can do from home; just click on virtual volunteering to find out more). Here are some big and small ideas to mull over; choose one of these, or brainstorm other ideas that resonate with you (see the Resources section for many website links):

- **Become a bilingual mentor.** If you speak two languages, why not offer to help others who are getting their footing in a new language?

- **Volunteer for disaster relief.** Check out the Red Cross or other local agencies that focus on crisis relief.

- **Become a host family for an international student.** Offer your home to a young student planning to study in the U.S. There is a good chance the relationship you develop could last for decades.

- **Become a volunteer crisis counselor via text.** Committing a few hours a week to respond to texts of someone in a mental health crisis is invaluable (https://www.crisistextline.org).

- **Deliver food to a senior or family in need.** If you have a car and a big heart, delivering food can be life-saving (try Meals on Wheels).

- **Volunteer at a local senior residence.** Many seniors feel alone and isolated; a friendly visit can make all the difference to their day. Attend a volunteer orientation to see if this is a fit.

- **Volunteer at a veterans' hospital or home.** If you have a soft spot in your heart for veterans (like I do, since my father was a veteran and I worked at a VA hospital for many years), check out your community veterans hospital's volunteer service and see what they may need (visit https://volunteer.va.gov).

- **Volunteer at an animal shelter.** All animal shelters could use your helping hand to care for their animals, is this where your heart is? (The Humane Society is one to try.)

- **Foster kittens or cats, puppies or dogs.** If you have the room in your home and the time needed to foster animals, why not look into it?

- **Volunteer for a cause near to your heart.** There are many medical causes that need extra help; find one that you connect with and reach out to them.

- **Help children learn to read.** Some children have had a rough go over the past few years, and many are behind in reading. Giving a bit of your time to this can change a kid's life for the long run (visit https://help2read.org).

- **Engage in community arts.** Providing singing or art lessons in a community center may be just the ticket to lift someone's spirit and your own.

- **Provide your time to help with environmental causes.** A neighborhood can be reborn if you help build a home, plant trees, or help clean up a park, a beach, or a whole block (you could start with Habitat for Humanity).

- **Give your time to a local women's shelter.** Assisting women as they make the important transitions in their lives will have a lasting impact. If this is your passion, don't hesitate to reach out to a shelter in your area.

- **Serve food at a homeless shelter.** Shelters are always looking for volunteers, especially around the holidays. Make a commitment to see what is needed in your local area.

- **Connect with your local food bank.** Food banks help millions of people find food and groceries in their communities each year. Is this something that sparks your interest? (Try the Feeding America website.)

- **Help a local business with your social media skills.** If you're lucky enough to be great at social media, chances are many of your neighborhood businesses are not and could use your help (Volunteer Match usually has positions like this).

As you can see, there are countless volunteer opportunities waiting for someone just like you. Letting go of alcohol may offer you more time for giving back. Even if you offer just a few hours a week, it will make a big difference in someone's life, in an animal's life, or in the life of a community. And it will make a big difference in your life too!

50. Find Joy in Everyday Moments

Little moments of joy are there for you every day. It's all about being available to notice them. When you move ahead with a nondrinking lifestyle, you get to see what else there is to be joyful for.

Joy is not something you can grab and hold on tight to. Joy is the experience of an open hand and an open heart. Joy is the experience of connecting with yourself and with others. There is no single right way to be joyful; there is only your way.

You might be surprised how easy it is to start a joy practice—and how your practice will boost your mood, improve your health, and make your days just a little bit lighter. Here are a few simple ways to explore your joy every day; choose one to try this week:

- **Change your focus.** Instead of focusing on the gloom and doom of the news or the next bad thing that is about to happen, focus on small joyful moments. Smile at someone at the store, give an unexpected compliment, listen to the rain, laugh with a child, or notice the change of seasons.

- **Send out positive energy.** If you know someone who is having a hard time, let them know that you're thinking about them and sending them love. This tiny joy practice is good for both of you.

- **Breathe in joy, breathe out stress.** As you know, I'm a believer in the power of conscious breathing to calm the nervous system and lead to moments of deep peace, reflection, and joy. This is something you can return to any time of day for a little boost of lightness.

- **This very moment.** Look around you right here and now. What do you see, feel, hear, and sense? Could this be your joyful moment? Give a quiet thanks for everything that has brought you to this moment.

● ● ● ● ●

Take a few minutes now to honestly answer these questions about uplifting your spirit:

What can I offer my spirit today?

What can I let go of to serve my spirit today?

Celebrate Your Spirit Checklist

You have a special opportunity here to celebrate your integrity, who you are, and how you're interacting with the world. Take a look at this checklist and choose one area you'd like to focus your energy on this week:

- ☐ Give yourself one opportunity to rebalance in the here and now.

- ☐ Choose one way to get your art on.

- ☐ Find one like-minded person you can reach out to and offer support or receive support.

- ☐ Find one way to give a little back to your community.

- ☐ Notice a few moments of joy in the everyday.

I'm so impressed that you've walked this path with me of intentionally changing your relationship with alcohol. By choosing ways to unwind without alcohol, you've custom designed a practice that is a perfect fit for you right now. In the weeks and months ahead, return to the lists of suggestions here to add new ways to unwind that you haven't tried yet. Keep going and embrace all that this stunning life has to offer you. Congratulations, my friend!

Notes of Gratitude

There is always a tribe that surrounds an artist and the art she produces. I've been lucky to have such a tribe during my writing journey. For twelve years and counting, the team at New Harbinger has been that tribe for me.

I send out the warmest thank-you to Jennye Garibaldi, my unstoppable acquisitions editor, for her patience, kindness, and inspiration. She guides her writers with compassion and clarity. Jennye offers the unconditional support that all writers need to develop and create.

I offer profound gratitude to the editorial skills of Madison Davis, the art direction of Amy Shoup, the marketing expertise of Analis Souza, the business acumen of Safa Shokrai, the foreign rights expertise of Dorothy Smyk and Katie Parr, the campaign management of Ifeoma Odiwe, and the copyediting insights of Kristi Hein.

My love and appreciation travels across the pond to Beth Kempton, my writing teacher in England. Her writing courses kept me in the flow during challenging times. Rick Rubin's book, *The Creative Act: A Way of Being*, gave me a surprise spiritual lift as I rounded the corner on this project.

I send a heartfelt note of gratitude to Julie Kraft, my writing partner of over a decade. Although this book is a solo writing adventure, I loved working with Julie on our two collaborations: *The Gift of Recovery: 52 Mindful Ways to Live Joyfully Beyond Addiction* and *The Mindfulness Workbook for Addiction: A Guide to Coping with the Grief, Stress, and Anger That Trigger Addictive Behaviors*, now happily in its second edition.

Last, but certainly not least, I thank my husband, Michael. All of my thinking, daydreaming, and creating would not be possible without your love, laughter, and everlasting support. Honey, this book is your book too.

Resources

Body

Dalton-Smith, S. *Sacred Rest: Recover Your Life, Renew Your Energy, and Restore Your Sanity*. Brentwood, TN: Faith Words Publishing, 2017.

Stanley, T. *Radiant Rest: Yoga Nidra for Deep Relaxation and Awakened Clarity*. Boulder, CO: Shambala, 2021.

Streets, A. *52 Ways to Walk: The Surprising Science of Walking for Wellness and Joy, One Week at a Time*. New York: G. P. Putnam's Sons, 2022.

Yogafinder.com: https://yogafinder.com.

Family

Schonbrun, Y. *Work, Parent, Thrive: 12 Science-Backed Strategies to Ditch Guilt, Manage Overwhelm, and Grow Connection (When Everything Feels Like Too Much)*. Boulder, CO: Shambala, 2022.

Food and Drink

Barefoot Contessa: https://barefootcontessa.com/search/results?q=vegetarian.

Branson, B. *Seedlip Cocktails: 100 Delicious Nonalcoholic Recipes from Seedlip & The World's Best Bars*. San Francisco: Weldon Owen, 2020.

DeAngelis, D. "Our 20 Most Popular Vegetarian Recipes of 2022. *Eating Well*. https://www.eatingwell.com/gallery/8018874/best-vegetarian-recipes-of-2022. December 14, 2022.

EatingWell: https://www.eatingwell.com/recipes/18005/lifestyle-diets/vegetarian.

Food Network: https://www.foodnetwork.com.

Food Safety: https://www.foodsafety.gov/food-safety-charts.

Giadzy: https://giadzy.com/search?q=healthyveggies#recipes.

Happy Cow: https://www.happycow.net.

Licalzi, D., and K. Benson. *Mocktail Party: 75 Plant-Based, Non-Alcoholic Mocktail Recipes for Every Occasion*. Bend, OR: Blue Star Press, 2021.

Recipes.com: https://www.recipes.com.

Sober Bars Near Me: https://soberbarsnearme.com.

Taylor, K. *Love Real Food: More Than 100 Feel-Good Vegetarian Favorites to Delight the Senses and Nourish the Body: A Cookbook*. Emmaus, PA: Rodale, 2017.

Health and Well-Being

American Massage Therapy Association: https://www.amtamassage.org/resources/massage-and-health.

Gaiam TV Fit & Yoga: https://www.gaia.com/lp/gaiamtv.

Mindful.org. "Loving-Kindness Meditation with Sharon Salzberg." https://www.mindful.org/loving-kindness-meditation-with-sharon-salzberg.

Home

Gill, S. *Minimalista: Your Step-by-Step Guide to a Better Home, Wardrobe, and Life*. Berkeley, CA: Ten Speed Press, 2021.

Kingston, K. *Clear Your Clutter with Feng Shui*. New York: Harmony, 2016.

Lembo, M. A. *The Essential Guide to Aromatherapy and Vibrational Healing*. Woodbury, MN: Llewellyn Publications, 2016.

Platt, C. *The Afrominimalist's Guide to Living with Less*. Easton, MD: Tiller Press. 2021.

The Spruce: https://www.thespruce.com.

Mind

Altman, D. *Clearing Emotional Clutter: Mindfulness Practices for Letting Go of What's Blocking Your Fulfillment and Transformation.* Novato, CA: New World Library, 2016.

Beattie, M. *Journey to the Heart: Daily Meditations on the Path to Freeing Your Soul.* San Francisco: HarperOne, 1996.

Chodron, P. *When Things Fall Apart: Heart Advice for Difficult Times.* Boulder, CO: Shambala, 2016.

Elle, A. *How We Heal: Uncover Your Power and Set Yourself Free.* San Francisco: Chronicle Books, 2022.

Price, C. *How to Break Up with Your Phone: The 30-Day Plan to Take Back Your Life.* Berkeley, CA: Ten Speed Press, 2018.

Money

Aliche, T. *Get Good with Money: Ten Simple Steps to Becoming Financially Whole.* Emmaus, PA: Rodale Books, 2021.

DeYoe, J. *Mindful Money: Simple Practices for Reaching Your Financial Goals and Increasing Your Happiness Dividend.* Novato, CA: New World Library, 2017.

Nerdwallet.com: https://www.nerdwallet.com/article/finance/tracking-monthly-expenses.

Thackray, G. *How to Manifest: Bring Your Goals into Alignment with the Alchemy of the Universe.* Berkeley, CA: Ten Speed Press, 2022.

Nature

Cheng, D. *New Plant Parent: Develop Your Green Thumb and Care for Your House-Plant Family.* New York: Abrams Image, 2019.

Coleman, M. *A Field Guide to Nature Meditations: 52 Mindfulness Practices for Joy, Wisdom, and Wonder.* Sausalito, CA: Awake in the Wild, 2022.

De La Paz, R. *Houseplants for Beginners: A Practical Guide to Choosing, Growing, and Helping Your Plants Thrive.* Emeryville, CA: Rockridge Press, 2021.

Netflix. *Moving Art.* https://www.netflix.com/title/80174902.

Relationships

Hanson, R. *Making Great Relationships: Simple Practices for Solving Conflicts, Building Connection, and Fostering Love.* New York: Harmony Books, 2023.

Lerner, H. *Why Won't You Apologize: Healing Big Betrayals and Everyday Hurts.* New York: Gallery Books, 2017.

Murphy, K. *You're Not Listening: What You're Missing and Why It Matters.* New York: Celadon Books, 2021.

Tawwab, N. G. *Set Boundaries, Find Peace: A Guide to Reclaiming Yourself.* New York: TarcherPerigee, 2021.

Spirit

Kempton, B. *The Way of the Fearless Writer: Ancient Eastern Wisdom for a Flourishing Writing Life.* London: Piatkus, 2022.

McKowen, L. *We Are the Luckiest: The Surprising Magic of a Sober Life.* Novato, CA: New World Library, 2022.

Rubin, R. *The Creative Act: A Way of Being.* New York: Penguin Press, 2023.

Williams, R. E., and J. S. Kraft. *The Gift of Recovery: 52 Mindful Ways to Live Joyfully Beyond Addiction.* Oakland, CA: New Harbinger Publications, 2018.

Volunteer Opportunities

Crisis Text Line: https://www.crisistextline.org/become-a-volunteer.

Habitat for Humanity: https://www.habitat.org/volunteer.

Help2Read.org: https://help2read.org/volunteer.

Humane Society: https://www.humanesociety.org/volunteer.

Meals on Wheels America: https://www.mealsonwheelsamerica.org.

Red Cross: https://www.redcross.org/volunteer/volunteer-role-finder.html.

Volunteer Match: https://www.volunteermatch.org.

VA Center for Development and Civic Engagement: https://volunteer.
va.gov.

Feeding America: https://www.feedingamerica.org/find-your-local-
foodbank.

Work

Brown, B. *Daring to Lead: Brave Work, Tough Conversations, Whole Hearts.*
New York: Random House, 2018.

Payscale: "Salary Negotiation Guide." https://www.payscale.com/salary-
negotiation-guide.

Salary: https://www.salary.com.

Salzberg, S. *Real Happiness at Work: Meditations for Accomplishment,
Achievement, and Peace.* New York: Workman, 2013.

Zetlin, M. *Career Self-Care: Find Your Happiness, Success, and Fulfillment at
Work.* Novato, CA: New World Library, 2022.

References

Acuff, S. F., J. C. Strickland, J. A. Tucker, and J. G. Murphy. 2022. "Changes in Alcohol Use During COVID-19 and Associations with Contextual and Individual Difference Variables: A Systematic Review and Meta-analysis." *Psychology of Addictive Behaviors*, 36(1): 1–19.

Benko, L. 2016. *Holistic Home: Feng Shui for Mind, Body, Spirit, and Space.* New York: Helios Press.

Boukes, M., and R. Vliegenthart. 2017. "News Consumption and Its Unpleasant Side Effect: Studying the Effect of Hard and Soft News Exposure on Mental Well-being over Time." *Journal of Media Psychology: Theories, Methods, and Applications* 29(3): 137–147.

Bratman, G. N., H. A. Olvera-Alvarez, and J. J. Gross. 2021. "The Affective Benefits of Nature Exposure." *Social and Personality Psychology Compass* 15(8): e12630. https://doi.org/10.1111/spc3.12630.

Capasso, A., A. M. Jones, S. H. Ali, J. Foreman, Y. Tozan, and R. J. DiClemente. 2021, April. "Increased Alcohol Use During the COVID-19 Pandemic: The Effect of Mental Health and Age in a Cross-sectional Sample of Social Media Users in the U.S." *Preventive Medicine* 145: 106422.

Chertoff, J. 2018. "What Are the Benefits of Walking? Plus Safety Tips and More." https://www.healthline.com/health/benefits-of-walking.

Chestney, K. 2020. *Radical Intuition: A Revolutionary Guide to Using Your Inner Power.* Novato, CA: New World Library.

Clifton, J., and J. Harter. 2021. *Wellbeing at Work: How to Build Resilient and Thriving Teams.* Washington, DC: Gallup Press.

Conrad, I. 2022. "Benefits of Massage Therapy." https://www.mayoclinichealthsystem.org/hometown-health/speaking-of-health/benefits-of-massage-therapy.

Ewert, C., A. Vater, and M. Schröder-Abé. 2021. "Self-compassion and Coping: A Meta-Analysis." *Mindfulness* 12: 1063–1077.

Geneshka, M., P. Coventry, J. Cruz, and S. Gilbody. 2021. "Relationship Between Green and Blue Spaces with Mental and Physical Health: A Systematic Review of Longitudinal Observational Studies." *International Journal of Environmental Research and Public Health* 18(17): 9010. https://doi.org/10.3390/ijerph18179010.

Gustavson, D. E., P. L. Coleman, J. R. Iversen, H. H. Maes, R. L. Gordon, and M. D. Lense. 2021. "Mental Health and Music Engagement: Review, Framework, and Guidelines for Future Studies." *Translational Psychiatry* 11: 370. https://doi.org/10.1038/s41398-021-01483-8.

Insurance Information Institute. 2022. "Facts + Statistics: Pet Ownership and Insurance." https://www.iii.org/fact-statistic/facts-statistics-pet-ownership-and-insurance.

Johns Hopkins Medicine. 2023. "9 Benefits of Yoga." Johnshopkinsmedicine.org. https://www.hopkinsmedicine.org/search?q=benefits+of+yoga.

Kwok, A., A. L. Dordevic, G. Paton, M. J. Page, and H. Truby. 2019. "Effect of Alcohol Consumption on Food Energy Intake: A Systematic Review and Meta-analysis." *British Journal of Nutrition* 121(5): 481–495. https://doi.org/10.1017/S0007114518003677.

Martela, F. 2020. *A Wonderful Life: Insights on Finding a Meaningful Existence*. New York: Harper Design Books.

Martin, L., S. Pahl, M. P. White, and J. May. 2019. "Natural Environments and Craving: The Mediating Role of Negative Affect." *Health & Place* 58: 102160. https://doi.org/10.1016/j.healthplace.2019.102160.

Martin, L., M. P. White, A. Hunt, M. Richardson, S. Pahl, and J. Burt. 2020. "Nature Contact, Nature Connectedness and Associations with Health, Well-being and Pro-environmental Behaviours." *Journal of Environmental Psychology* 68: 101389. https://doi.org/10.1016/j.jenvp.2020.101389.

Martin, M. 2022. "How to Ask Your Boss for a Raise: 5 Tips for Success." *Business News Daily*. https://www.businessnewsdaily.com/8101-asking-for-a-raise-tips.html.

Mayo Clinic. 2022. "Eyestrain." https://www.mayoclinic.org/diseases-conditions/eyestrain/diagnosis-treatment/drc-20372403.

Mayo Clinic. 2023 "Vegetarian Diet: How to Get the Best Nutrition." https://www.mayoclinic.org/healthy-lifestyle/nutrition-and-healthy-eating/in-depth/vegetarian-diet/art-20046446.

Meija, Z., and R. T. Spann. 2022. "10 Science-Backed Benefits of Meditation." https://www.forbes.com/health/mind/benefits-of-meditation.

National Council on Aging. 2021. "10 Reasons Why Hydration is Important." https://ncoa.org/article/10-reasons-why-hydration-is-important.

National Institutes of Health (NIH). 2023. "Good Hydration Linked to Healthy Aging." https://irp.nih.gov/news-and-events/in-the-news/good-hydration-linked-to-healthy-aging.

Oliver, M. 2020. *Devotions: The Selected Poems of Mary Oliver*. New York: Penguin Publishing Group.

Pollock, M. M., R. E. Williams, and S. M. Gomez. 2017. "Animals as Icebreakers: A Pilot Animal-Assisted Therapy Group for Veterans with Serious Mental Illness." *International Journal of Psychosocial Rehabilitation* 21(1): 123–135.

Raheem, O. 2022. *Pause, Rest, Be: Stillness Practices for Courage in Times of Change*. Boulder, CO: Shambala Publications.

Salzberg, S. 2018. *LovingKindness: The Revolutionary Art of Happiness*. Boulder, CO: Shambala Publications.

Silver, N. 2020. "16 Reasons Why Water Is Important to Human Health." https://www.healthline.com/health/food-nutrition/why-is-water-important.

Terry, B. 2020. *Vegetable Kingdom: The Abundant World of Vegan Recipes*. Berkeley, CA: Ten Speed Press.

Walia, N., J. Matas, A. Turner, S. Gonzalez, and R. Zoorob. 2021. "Yoga for Substance Abuse: A Systemic Review." *The Journal of the American Board of Family Medicine*, 35(5): 964–973.

Young-Mason, J. 2020. "Nature Documentaries: An Antidote to Anxiety and Fear in the Time of COVID-19 Pandemic." *Clinical Nurse Specialist* 34(4): 182–183. https://doi.org/10.1097/NUR.0000000000000526.

About the Author

Rebecca E. Williams, **PhD**, is a psychologist, wellness expert, and award-winning author. She received her bachelor's degree from Williams College; her master's degree from Harvard; and her doctorate with a specialization in clinical psychology from the University of California, Santa Barbara. Rebecca enjoyed a twenty-year career as a clinic director with the San Diego VA Healthcare System; was an associate clinical professor in the School of Medicine at the University of California, San Diego; and maintained an active private practice. She is coauthor of two popular books bridging addiction recovery with the power of mindfulness. *The Gift of Recovery* is a "pocket coach" designed to strengthen recovery. *The Mindfulness Workbook for Addiction* is a go-to guide for understanding the relationship between moods and substance use. The workbook is now in its second edition, and has been translated into multiple languages. Her website is www.mindfulnessworkbook.com.

Real change *is* possible

For more than forty-five years, New Harbinger has published proven-effective self-help books and pioneering workbooks to help readers of all ages and backgrounds improve mental health and well-being, and achieve lasting personal growth. In addition, our spirituality books offer profound guidance for deepening awareness and cultivating healing, self-discovery, and fulfillment.

Founded by psychologist Matthew McKay and Patrick Fanning, New Harbinger is proud to be an independent, employee-owned company. Our books reflect our core values of integrity, innovation, commitment, sustainability, compassion, and trust. Written by leaders in the field and recommended by therapists worldwide, New Harbinger books are practical, accessible, and provide real tools for real change.

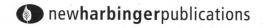 **newharbinger**publications

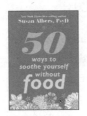
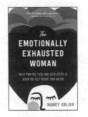
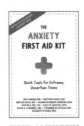
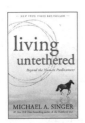
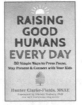
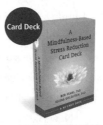